THE
HEARTBREAK
OF STILLBIRTH

One Mother's Story of Loss, Grief,
& Learning to Live Again

AMANDA DUNN

©2013 Amanda Dunn

All rights reserved. No portion of this book may be reproduced, stored in a retrieval system, or transmitted in any form or by any means—electronic, mechanical, photocopy, recording, or any other—except for brief quotations in printed reviews, without the prior permission of the publisher.

Scriptures taken from the Holy Bible, New International Version®, NIV®. Copyright © 1973, 1978, 1984, 2011 by Biblica, Inc.™ Used by permission of Zondervan. All rights reserved worldwide. www.zondervan.com The "NIV" and "New International Version" are trademarks registered in the United States Patent and Trademark Office by Biblica, Inc.™

Editing: Nina Taylor
For help with your book project, contant Nina at nina.g.taylor@gmail.com.

ISBN: 978-0-9892776-0-0

To my husband Christian:
One day we will hold them again. Until then,
may we cling to one another.

And to my children:
My love for each one of you is unquenchable.

Contents

FOREWORD		vii
ACKNOWLEDGEMENTS		ix
INTRODUCTION		1
CHAPTER 1	The Day That Changed Our Lives Forever	9
CHAPTER 2	The Birth	23
CHAPTER 3	Leaving	35
CHAPTER 4	Back to Normal	43
CHAPTER 5	Surprised by Hope	57
CHAPTER 6	My Battle with Mental Anguish	77
CHAPTER 7	Freedom to Grieve	93
CHAPTER 8	Letting Your Children Grieve	101
CHAPTER 9	Grieving Together	113
CHAPTER 10	"Trying Again"	125
CHAPTER 11	A Gift, Not a Substitute	139

Foreword

There are some stories that take our breath away — that stun us and remind us of the fragility of life. So it is with Mandy Dunn's story. As her pastor, I had a close-up view of the grief and prolonged times of great pain she experienced while saying good-bye to one stillborn child, and then, shockingly, another. As a professional counselor, I am trained to remain objective and in control of my emotions, but Mandy's story gripped me on a personal level. I hated to see her walk through a darkness that only a select few ever experience. I never wanted her to be a part of that particular club. However, Mandy can now write about the dark night of the soul with the sort of authority and sincerity one can only gain from having first been there. And that's what makes this book so special.

    As a counselor, I know what it looks like to watch someone in crisis. While there, we are presented with choices that either usher in healing, or prolong the suffering. We make decisions to either tough it out— doggedly walking on our own while refusing any help from others — or we choose to stay in community, allowing others to walk alongside us, taking in kindness and comfort and counsel. Mandy has had overlapping crises to walk through, and she has made healing choices along the way. She stayed in community while everything in her wanted to just be alone and grieve her losses. She sought out professional help, admitting that she couldn't get through this time in her life on her own. She asked for prayer again and again and again. She was honest with God and was willing to voice the hard questions. And she wrote her story down.

The details of our individual stories differ, but the themes are what tie us together as people. We all suffer. We all hope. We all know bitter disappointment. And we all want to feel better. It is important to relay our hurts and just as important to relay how we healed. To describe the beauty we saw from the bottom of the pit of despair. To talk about the first time we laughed again, after we'd sworn our days of joy had been replaced with a bitterness to rival the Pacific Ocean. When we are reeling from pain, we need to know that we are not the only ones to feel loss. We are comforted by others who have gone before us, who have cried tears that no mother should, and yet have continued to live, to walk with grace, to care for others, to laugh, to make jokes, and even to carry hope within them again — because that hope becomes a sort of lighthouse. And when we are lost in the storm, we look up and see the lighthouse in the distance; we decide that, eventually, we will make it to land, too.

Mandy's story is a lighthouse. The words in 2 Corinthians are brought to life in her journey: "God comforts us in all our troubles so that we can then comfort those in any trouble with the comfort we ourselves have received from God."

Rev. Lynn Latshaw, M.C.

Acknowledgments

This book would not have been possible without the love and support of so many people. I would like to give special thanks to:

 My friend and editor Nina Taylor. Thank you for your countless hours of work, and for making my words make sense. You are a miracle worker!

 My church family and pastors. Your outpouring of love and support has blown me away. Thank you for holding my family in your arms and prayers.

 My close friends (you know who you are!). Thank you for encouraging me to write even when my words failed me.

 My father-and mother-in-law, Brad and Jan Dunn. Your kindness, generosity, and love are evident to all. Thank you for extending your love to me time and time again. I am honored to have you in my life.

 My parents, Charles and Laurie Wendell, and Christine Beattie, and my grandmother Betty Wendell. God has allowed me to have such incredible parents. Many children do not have one loving parent such as you, and I was blessed with unending love and support! Thank you each for wrapping your arms around me in the darkest times of my life.

THE HEARTBREAK OF STILLBIRTH

My brothers-in-law, Jonathan Latshaw and Alex Duzan, for your support, love, counsel, and friendship. I am so grateful to have godly men like you in my life, and in the lives of my children.

My sisters and best friends, Heather Duzan and Rebekah Latshaw. I don't know where I would be without you. As I let my children go, you stood by me in every way possible. You gave, even in your grief. You have listened and loved unconditionally. Thank you doesn't come close to the unconditional love you each pour upon me as you continue to walk with me.

To my husband Christian. I am truly overwhelmed by your love for me. You stood by me when I was shattered into a million pieces. Unable to put me back together, you sat with me, held my hand, and loved me in my brokenness. Thank you for holding me up even when you could barely stand. I love you more every day.

Introduction

If you would have told me nearly six years ago that I would write a book, well, I would have laughed right in your face. I am not a writer. My grammar, spelling, and lack of creative vocabulary are horrendous! I am often amazed at my inability to lay out my thoughts on paper or, in this case, on the computer. Writing a book would never have crossed my mind. Writing books is for extremely intelligent and creative people. Don't worry — I am not putting myself down. I know I am smart. I know I am creative. But I also know I'm not off the chart in either of those categories. I am just average. I am okay with average.

Isn't it funny how God seems to always find a way to give us the motivation and strength in an area of our lives, when we didn't even know it was possible? That is pretty much what happened with this book. I was in the darkest place in my life and had nowhere to go. Going to God wasn't always comfortable either. So, I wrote.

I found myself pouring out my heart in ridiculously long e-mails to my sisters and closest friends about losing my son Malachi. He died in my third trimester of pregnancy with no clear reason to blame. He was stillborn.

THE HEARTBREAK OF STILLBIRTH

A year later, I found myself feeling even more claustrophobic with the death of our daughter Hope. She too died in the third trimester of an unknown cause. She too was stillborn.

I had nowhere else to go. I would find myself awake at night, mourning, and all I could do at times was write. How ironic. The one thing I never thought I would do is all that could "help" me at the darkest hour. I could vent and it was a safe place with people that loved me; at least I wasn't suffering alone. Someone out there knew what I was feeling and was praying.

I knew my sisters and my friends couldn't change, fix, or even lessen my load of grief. But the idea though that I could lay all my dirty laundry out there and there was no judgment was somehow therapeutic. So, that is what I did. I wrote and wrote and wrote.

I also wondered, what do people do who don't have the support I have? I began to toss around the idea of sharing my pain outside my network of family and close friends. What did that look like to me? It isn't like me to share my heart with everyone. I am an open gal, but when it comes to certain things, I like privacy. Sharing how I felt meant being vulnerable in a place that was raw and fragile. Places I don't want everyone knowing about. Places that I don't want people's opinions. Places that are close to sacred. Why would I do this to myself?

The answer that came isn't really profound or magical. It is simple: God wanted me to. I felt Him leading me to somehow put all these e-mails and thoughts together. So, that is exactly what I did.

Of course, because I have many opinions and a big mouth, once I started to put the pages in order, I had more to say about certain issues. It began as my "story" of losing our children, and it still is that. But it also became what we have learned on this journey. For a girl with only basic grammar knowledge and a suffering vocabulary, suddenly I had a ton to

Introduction

say and those small matters didn't hinder me. That's when you know it is God.

I make it sound so easy. Like it all just fell together. I wish that had been the case. This book has literally been soaked in tears. Well, my computer keyboard has been anyway. It has been an emotional journey I never expected to take.

First and foremost I have written this book as an act of obedience to God. Secondly, I have written this book in memory of my adorable son Malachi and my beautiful daughter Hope. My love for them goes beyond the grave.

My desire is that this book touches the places in your heart where you need to hear that you are not alone. We all suffer in this world. We cling to the promise that there will be a day when our Father in heaven will restore everything. A verse my husband was given from God when our daughter Hope died was from Isaiah 43: 5-7. The whole chapter is amazing but the verses that stick out for me are:

> Do not be afraid for I am with you:
> I will bring your children from the east and
> Gather you from the west.
>
> I will say to the north, "Give them up!"
> And to the south, " Do not hold them back!"
> Bring my sons from afar and my daughters from the
> Ends of the earth.
>
> Everyone who is called by my name,
> Whom I created for my glory
> Whom I formed and made.

THE HEARTBREAK OF STILLBIRTH

In this world we will suffer. However, we have a Redeemer — the One who will be true to His living Word, the One who knows there will be a day when He will "wipe every tear from [our] eyes" (Revelation 7:17).

Until that amazing day when we are all restored with the ones who have gone before us, I pray this book will bring you comfort. I know it won't change your "story." I know it won't lessen your travel load, but I pray the Lord uses this book in a way to let you know you are not alone.

We cried a lot tonight. Death seems so real now. Christian is heartbreaking when he cries. I get these times to see his sorrow and it pains me. He was talking tonight about how he had so many plans for Malachi and how he was so excited to teach one more little one all the things he has taught our three living children.

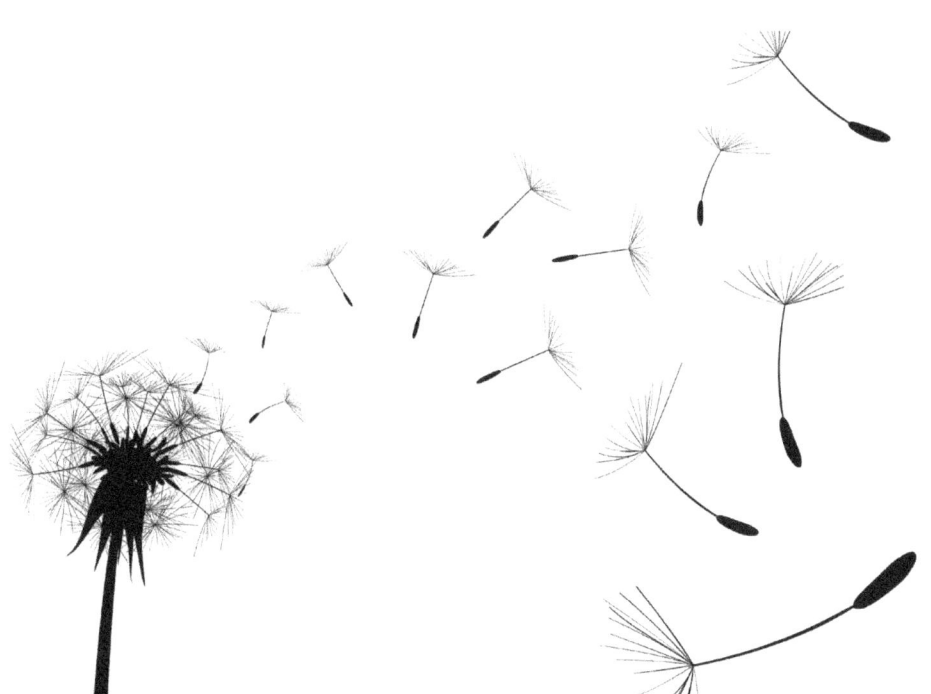

1

The Day That Changed Our Lives Forever

It was July 28, 2006, and I was headed to the birth center for my routine appointment. That morning I really wanted my family to come with me, but my appointment was at 9 a.m. and getting all three kids ready on what was supposed to be my husband's relaxing day off seemed too rushed. I kept thinking, *"Just ask Christian [my husband] to get the kids all ready and he will make it happen."* But every time I went to ask him, I found myself completely mute. I couldn't say it. Of course, now I know the Lord knew better. He knew what was about to take place, and He was already covering our children.

With every one of our children I made it a practice to lay my hand upon my belly and pray for the baby on the way to my appointments. But this time I never prayed. I felt led to turn on Keith Green's song, "Oh Lord, You're Beautiful." I was trying not to cry, but my emotions overwhelmed me. I then listened to "Open the Eyes of My Heart" and "Let it Rain" by Michael W. Smith. Looking back I remember thinking that I hadn't felt any movement, but I just thought the baby was asleep. It was a passing thought really.

Having carried three children to full term, I had experienced quiet days before. I wasn't alarmed. Oh, but looking back, Thursday evening was quiet and I fell asleep early. In the middle of the night a huge thunderstorm came bolting through. Trees came down throughout the neighborhood and we lost power for three hours. My sister Rebekah later shared with me that she felt it was the Lord showing His anger at Malachi's death — letting us know that He hates death and all that it brings.

When I arrived at the birth center, it was talk as usual, including talk of my older sister, Heather, who had delivered her son that very week — three days prior to my appointment. There was also talk of my gaining nine pounds in a month! This was my usual gain for this time of pregnancy. My belly was even a few days ahead of schedule. It was the first time I was measured during this pregnancy. I was so excited to be getting bigger and showing more. My belly was in full force and I was so happy to be pregnant.

Then the midwife began to listen for the heartbeat . . .

She couldn't find one.

So she changed the probe to the early trimester probe, hoping that was all we needed. She said the probe acted up sometimes. Yet she still couldn't find the heartbeat. There was a glimmer of hope — we both looked at each other as if we had heard a few rushed, swooshing beats — but that faded in an instant. I told the midwife, "This is stressing me out!" She went out to get the head midwife, whom we have known for years, to have her try to find the heartbeat.

She came in very upbeat asking, "Is this little peanut hiding from us?" I could barely speak. Her face seemed so hopeful — but where was the heartbeat?

I could see the growing concern on her face as soon as she started to listen. Her smile slowly faded and her hope-filled voice turned serious.

The Day that Changed Our Lives Forever

She asked for the stethoscope to attach it to the Doppler. I began to cry. I lay there as I watched her scan every inch of my belly and I just cried. I knew. This was all wrong. I was too far along for it to take this long. Even early on it never took this long to find a heartbeat. She called the secretary in to hold my hand while she kept trying to listen. In tears I said, "I haven't felt the baby move since I have been laying here!" She had the other midwife making calls to find a place to have an ultrasound. I was in total shock.

They sent me to the back room to wait and to call Christian. He could hear in my voice that something was wrong. He sounded panicked, "What's wrong?!"

I burst into tears, "They can't find the baby's heartbeat!"

He said, "I am on my way."

My sister went over and watched our kids and Christian met me about forty-five minutes later at the maternity triage at the hospital. Before I left the birthing center, the midwife asked if she could listen one more time. I got on the table, praying that this would all go away and that we would hear the heartbeat. There was no heartbeat to be found. She said, "Mandy, this is very concerning. I don't want to sound hopeless. Let's not give up hope, but this isn't good."

She insisted on driving me to the hospital, but in all my shock I told her I would drive myself. I kept telling her some nonsense about needing the car seats. As if I couldn't ever get them again. I was just in shock. I remember saying out loud in my car, "I can't do this Lord… I can't do this." And I wondered to myself: whose life am I leading? Maybe this is awful to say, but even though I should have had hope, I had none. My heart was vacant. I am not sure if it was all the confusion and shock or if it was my heart knowing we had lost our baby.

There was paperwork to do when we arrived. Our midwife sat

THE HEARTBREAK OF STILLBIRTH

with me trying to soothe me by talking about our three children at home. I kept looking for Christian, "When will he get here?" I needed him to be with me. I kept thinking I heard footsteps, but I had to wait. I needed my husband. I needed him to hold me and to tell me he could change it all. That everything would be fine. I needed him to just be with me.

I sat there filling out all of the forms and watching other pregnant women walk through going to their appointments. They had smiles on their faces and were excited to go to their visit. I remember looking at them with such despair. Their babies were alive.

I was taken to a room to be dressed for the ultrasound. I was in the bathroom dressing into a gown when I heard his sweet voice — the man I am so thankful that I married. I couldn't wait to get dressed. We hugged and he just held me so tightly, asking me if I was alright and how I was doing. I could see his stress-filled eyes. He was in distress. I was crying and he was being thrown into this just as I had been. I lay there waiting for the doctor and the ultrasound machine. It was the cursory ultrasound. Apparently, it gives an overview while you wait for the wet ultrasound to be taken. It was efficient enough to look for the baby's heartbeat or to detect any movement.

The time had come. The gel was cold and the room was quiet. Christian grabbed my hand and squeezed it. We waited for what seemed like hours. I could only see the side of the screen but I knew the baby wasn't moving. His little body just lay still in my womb. I watched, wanting to see his heart beating but knowing that it wouldn't be. The doctor said, "I am so sorry, there is no heartbeat or fetal movement. I am so sorry."

I began to weep.

Christian made a groaning sound, stood up from his chair and lifted my upper body up from the bed and held me. He and I just cried.

The Day that Changed Our Lives Forever

Those deep tears that come from the very core of who you are. We held each other and mourned our child.

Our midwife, who had come to the hospital and was in the room with us, cried as well. She had delivered two of our three children and cared for us through the years, so this was painful for her too. The doctor said that he would run one more ultrasound to make sure and then take it from there. I am not sure why he wanted to do this; it may have had something to do with the machine he had just used. Again we waited.

A few minutes later we were taken to the ultrasound room where the technician was waiting for us. She looked stressed and uneasy. I think she had been prepped as to why we were there. We sat in that dark room watching her scan my belly and again we saw no movement. She looked at us and with a tear stained face she said, "I am so sorry." She asked us if we wanted to know the gender. We had never made the choice with our other kids to find out the gender before they were born. In this situation we now realized we did want to find out before I had to deliver the baby. We wanted to be able to tell the kids the gender as well. She then told us what I felt I already knew….it was a boy. We cried so hard. It was Malachi. We had been holding this name in our hearts for some time, and he was finally here, but we would not get to have him for long here on this earth.

The technician left the room apologizing and saying that she was unprofessional for crying. We kept telling her that it was fine and that we appreciated her sadness. She came back a few minutes later and asked us if we wanted some pictures of him from the ultrasound. Of course we wanted anything that we could have of him. The doctor who reads the ultrasounds then came in and confirmed yet again that Malachi was not alive.

We then were carted back to the room. I felt like I was on display, as if all eyes were on me. I am sure that everyone knew what was going on with us. I just wanted to escape it all somehow. We got back to our room, and the doctor proceeded to tell us what would need to take place for delivery. Christian couldn't grasp the idea that I would have to deliver him. For some reason I think we both thought they would give me a C-section, but they informed us that this wasn't the case. I would have to deliver him naturally. Christian just shook his head and I kept hearing him sigh these deep sighs. The doctor said that we could take a few days to come back if we desired to do so.

We decided fairly quickly that we would come back the next day and deliver him. We both felt that it wouldn't be fair to the kids to have them waiting several days. I couldn't fathom watching them kiss my belly each day (as they always did) and trying to explain that he had died. I didn't want any of us to have to go through that for days. So we made the proper arrangements and started on our way home.

Telling and Retelling the Bad News
As we left the hospital, we cried. We were in shock. How did this day turn out like this? It started out so normally. How did we get to this place? We called my sister Rebekah first. I knew she was around our kids so I asked her to go upstairs so I could talk to her. I could tell from her voice that she already knew what I was about to say. I then told her, "We lost him." She just wept and all I could hear was her awful broken cry. Her heart was broken for me. She told me how sorry she was and that she would do anything for me that we needed. I told her that we were on our way home and that we would tell our kids when we got home. She would then have to go home and tell her kids as well.

I then called my older sister, Heather. I felt so badly telling her because she had just delivered her son three days earlier. When I told her, she too wept. She just felt awful — her sadness was so evident. She would now have to tell her children. It is so sad that all the cousins were so excited to see and hold their new friend and now it would never be. I felt so much pain for them all. My sisters and all of our children are so close; I knew this would be so much for them all to go through.

I got to the place where I couldn't call anyone anymore. I just couldn't do it. We made a few more calls, and then we had to quickly figure out what we were going to tell our children. Whenever it started to sound like we had the words, we would cry and know that no matter what we said….this was going to break their hearts.

Telling our kids that Malachi had died was beyond compare to anything I have ever had to explain. There just aren't words to explain death to little ones. I myself felt confused about what was happening. I guess I could have just said, "We live in a fallen world…life stinks…get used to it." Or, I could have said, "God picks who He wants to live here and He didn't pick Malachi." I am obviously being sarcastic here because there just aren't words. There isn't a manual that comes with life and tragedy. . How do you answer your children honestly when you do not know the answers? They are little and they expect us to have some clue about why things happen. But we were thrust into this situation as much as they were and we didn't feel like we had any answers.

When we walked in the door, they could tell something was wrong. But they had just had pizza with their cousins and they were happy. They had no real idea what had taken place. All they knew was that the doctors had to check the baby because there might be something wrong. As children they simply understood this as, "Oh, I get sick and doctors check me out…everything will be fine." They had no idea what was coming their way.

We called them over to us and we told them that the baby had gotten very sick inside my belly — not the kind of sickness that a Mommy or Daddy can see because the baby is inside. And it wasn't the kind of sickness that they could become sick with. The baby got so sick that the only way for him to feel better was for Jesus to take him to heaven and heal him there.

We told them that it wasn't Mommy's fault. Mommy couldn't see the baby to know that he was sick. We told them that they had done nothing wrong — that Malachi dying wasn't their fault either. (This seems obvious to us as adults, but you never know how kids will internalize this kind of tragedy, and we wanted to be careful.) We also expressed that we loved them so much and we were so thankful for each of them. We told them that they brought us so much joy. We tried to explain that we were going to be sad and cry a lot. We also said that other people they knew and loved were going to be sad and cry too. We just plainly told them that we were sad because he had died. It was okay for them if they were sad that Malachi had died. It was okay to be sad. It was fine to cry. It was also fine if they didn't want to cry. We wanted them to know that they didn't have to cry or be sad if they didn't want too. We told them that we knew they missed Malachi even if they didn't cry.

After telling them the baby had died, we told them that the baby was a boy. We never find out the gender of our babies before they are born, this was eventful news for them. They then said things like, "Mommy, Malachi isn't dead. He is still in your belly. I can see him in there." My belly was still big and they understood this concept. So we had to explain that yes, he was still in there but his spirit was in heaven. Imagine that one! I mean, try to explain to little kids that your baby has died, he is still in your belly because his body is there, yet he is in heaven!

How confusing is that for a kid? We told them that it is like when you ask Jesus into your heart. You don't see Him go in there but you know He is there because you asked Him to be in your heart. It was the same with Malachi. He had Jesus in his heart and his body would be here in Mommy because our bodies don't go to heaven, just our spirits. So Malachi's body was here but Malachi was already in heaven with Jesus.

They kept asking to kiss my belly and they wanted to lay on my belly. This was so difficult for me. I just wanted to lift them up off my belly and say, "He is dead. There is no reason to do this." But then I realized that they were saying good-bye. This was going to be the way that they got to say good-bye to their little brother. They wanted to let him know how much they would miss him. I then knew that this was so much bigger than just Christian and me. Our children were going to have to grieve. They had to do it in their own ways and not ours.

We told them that Malachi wasn't hurting anymore and that he was so happy to be with Jesus. We tried to explain as best we could that the person who gets to go to heaven isn't sad to leave this earth or their family. We tried to tell them that it is the people who are still here on the earth that are sad and cry. Malachi was so happy to feel better and to be with Jesus. Jesus was, and is, holding him and keeping him safe and Malachi loves to be with Him. He isn't afraid. We told them that Malachi wants to stay in heaven.

Of course this process of telling them was interrupted several times with questions. Some we had answers to and others we will not know until we get to heaven. They were so sad but their tears didn't come right away. I knew that they might not. They came much later — after the funeral and days after it had all set in. We were totally fine with this delay in outward emotion. We didn't want to force their hearts. They were already grieving, but they had to do it on their terms.

We had to explain that we weren't going to be home the next day because, "Mommy had to push out Malachi." Very raw to say, but that is how they understood it. They understood and knew that when I came back he would no longer be in my belly. That night we lay down with them as we put them to sleep. They all kissed my belly once more and told Malachi that they loved him and they would miss him. It was heart-wrenching to watch them let him go — seeing their little hands on my belly patting their brother and saying good-bye, talking to him one last time and letting him know that they would miss him. It was so unfair that they couldn't have their brother. They were so excited about him. They had these jobs that they wanted to do when he was born. Ways that they could help me out and help their brother. They had made their own plans for Malachi. Now, they had to let him go.

There wasn't much more we could do or say, we had to trust and pray that God would lead them the next day when we would not be home to comfort them.

What I Do Remember…
I don't remember much about that night. I can only recall that we cried and packed our bag. What a joke — — packing a bag. I mean that is the very bag that you are supposed to pack when you go and deliver your living baby. The bag that has all the stuff that will get you home with your little one. We even packed our camera. They had said that we might want to take pictures when he was born. I am so thankful that we did.

It was really late and we had to wake up early. But before we fall asleep at night we try to always read our Bible. I was reading a devotional book at the time and I turned to the page for that day. It was Psalm 139:13, "You created my inmost being; you knit me together in my mother's womb." I couldn't believe what I had read. Was God really speaking to me? Had He in my most desperate time already prepared for me to read this verse? Yes, He had. For the most part I was faithful in reading this devotional, but sometimes I would opt to read the Bible. It was so very evident that He wanted me to read this verse on this very night. He had saved this entry for me at this time. Even though the verse was almost tormenting to read, it also gave me comfort. God was letting me know that Malachi's inmost being was made whole and so was his earthly body. Even though my heart would not rest, his was no longer suffering. He was made perfect.

I feel like emotionally I have shut down. I can't allow myself to feel the total pain. When it hits me, it takes me over. I know I need to allow myself to go to that place . . . I guess I'm already here, but I don't want to open my eyes and look around. My surroundings in this place are dark and I cannot escape.

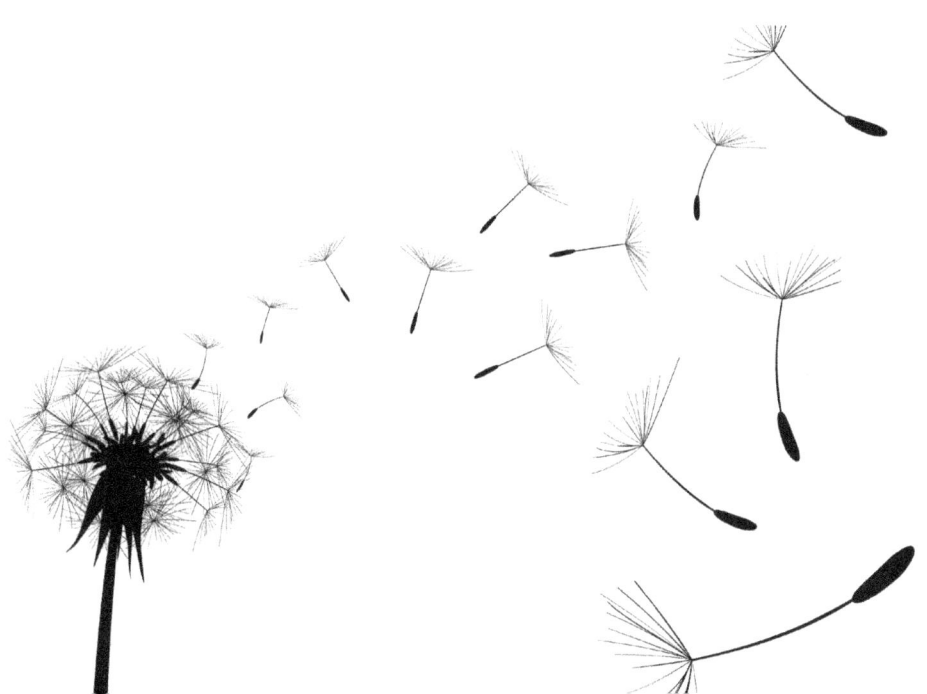

2

The Birth

Early in the morning we received a call from the hospital saying that we could come in. Everything there at the hospital was ready — everything but us. We arrived around 7 a.m. I couldn't stop crying. I just cried the whole trip up in the elevator. We walked in and there were little signs with pictures of baby feet showing moms and dads where to go in the hospital. These seemingly innocent signs tormented me.

I heard a baby cry as we walked the hallway. I could only cry more. Christian held my hand and we clung to one another. The nurse put us at the end of the hallway. It was the last room, away from all the noise and babies. She said that they would break all the rules for us. If we wanted tons of visitors, we could have them. If we wanted people to leave, she would make an excuse for them to go. She was going to try to do her best to make this as smooth as she could.

As we entered the room, it hit me — this is where he would be born. This is where we would say good-bye. I began to weep again. I couldn't hear anything more she had to say. She gave us some time and we cried. Being in that room felt like a mockery. Looking around and seeing all the pictures, colors, instruments — everything was designed to usher Malachi into this world living. This wasn't a room for suffering and loss. This was a room meant for life and joy.

When the nurse came back she explained the entire process to us. I was going to be induced and would need to continue to take the medication every four hours until labor was in full force. I chose not to have an epidural simply because I had never had one before. I was too afraid that my body would not connect with birth and I would be an outsider looking in. I only knew what to expect from natural childbirth. I was so emotional and such a wreck that I couldn't bring myself to have one. They offered the world as far as pain medication was concerned. But again, I was too afraid of what my body would do and how I would react. I needed to be connected with him as I was in my other births. That was the only way I knew, and given this situation I couldn't change anything. I even refused an IV. The nurse told me as long as my temperature didn't go up that I didn't have to have one. I think everything inside me wanted to be free from anything that connected me to losing him. Little did I know the physical pain wouldn't even come close to the emotional pain that was about to begin.

I knew full well that choosing against these medications meant going through the torture and exhaustion of labor, with no living baby as a reward at the end. Labor, especially natural childbirth, cannot be described in words. It is so painful, and it is not meant to be endured without the gift of your living baby as a reward. This, too, was a cruel mockery.

I was in that bed for two hours before the first dose, wanting to get the process started but knowing that it meant he would no longer be inside of me. The medicine was finally administered around 10:30 a.m. I remember lying there and holding the nurse's hand on one side and Christian's on the other. The attending resident asked me, "Are you

The Birth

ready?" I could barely speak. Ready for what? Ready to let my son go? No! I just wept. Everything within me wanted to refuse this medicine. I wanted to run far away from this hospital. I wanted to stop this horrific pain. I felt like such a bad mother. I felt that I was hurting Malachi, or that by doing this I was saying I was ready to let him go…

I knew this meant that the process of birth had begun. I had to lie there and wait for the medication to do its awful job. Making myself do this was such a struggle. I mean, I am allowing the very medicine to become effective that would take my son away from me. I had to choose to allow the pain to enter, and I felt like I was betraying my son. Like I was willingly letting him go. That just isn't what we do as parents — letting suffering happen to our children, knowing that you will be separated forever. I lay there because I had to, and it was the first step in letting him go.

They told us that it could take one to three days to deliver him. Each woman's body works so differently under induced labor. We just prayed that my body would respond and the medicine would be effective.

I began to feel the first signs of birth pains, but I knew that I wasn't close yet. Before too long, the second round of medication was administered. This round of medicine brought much more pain. A few hours into it, and I could feel the difference — my body was reacting more strongly. It wouldn't be too long before the intense labor would begin. We looked at each other and Christian once again held me and I cried. We knew that this meant Malachi was on his way.

I'll never forget being in labor and closing my eyes and telling my body that it had to let go of him. I could feel my body trying to hold on, raging against the medicine and trying to fight for him. We prayed and welcomed him into our arms just as we have prayed for all of our children. "It is safe here. We want to hold you, and it is time for you to be born." Those words I knew I couldn't completely understand until he was here — holding him and realizing that our arms would only hold him for a short while.

Throughout the labor, we had these times where we would look at each other and ask one another, "How are we ever going to get through this birth? How are we going to go through labor and delivery? How are we going to walk this out?" I knew Christian was so crushed and I knew that his pain was only going to increase.

Ready or Not . . .
The birth pains began to intensify around 5 p.m. that night. I remember we were trying to watch TV and take a break from our thoughts and emotions — trying to find some outlet, even if it was mindless TV. My sisters couldn't be there with us. At different times they had each come to the hospital to spend some time with us, but they couldn't stay all day. My older sister had just given birth three days prior to her son — their sixth child. My younger sister had an infant who was two-and-a-half months old and three other children. She was also helping care for our children. They wanted to be with us the entire time, but it was impossible. I cannot even begin to understand how difficult it must have been for them to leave me there. I could see the pain on their faces as they left. There was desperation in their eyes knowing what the next hours would hold for us. As sisters, we have an incredible bond. When they came to the hospital it felt so peaceful having them sitting with us. They never told me, but I know that they both cried the whole way home.

Because my sisters couldn't stay, one of my best friends, Darby, stayed with us. We have always said in life that we know we cannot replace our sisters (she has two as well), but we are the next best thing for each other if our sisters can't be with us. She stayed there and talked with

The Birth

us when it was quiet. She would leave when our families would come. When the pain was more than we could bear, she wept with us.

While she was there I felt my body begin to move into active labor. I told them that things were changing. Christian responded and he knew I was entering into the phase of labor where I would need his absolute attention. He was ready to carry me through.

I needed to walk around and let my body work with the contractions. The nurse checked me and I was only at 3 cm. The labor at this point felt like I was at 5 or 6 cm. I went to the bathroom again and I was just standing in there and praying to God and asking Him to help me. I told Malachi that we loved him so much and it was time for him to be born. We welcomed him into our family and told him it was time to come and that it was safe. I asked God to give me strength to give birth. I felt the panic start to set in. I knew that this would all be over within a few hours and I was terrified of it being over.

Mentally, I tried to place myself at the birth center where we had delivered our other three children. I tried to flow with the contractions. Those birthing pains were so very painful in every way. Physically, my body was trying to let him go, but my heart was holding on. It was a brutal mind game. I was in so much pain after laboring for a few hours. I think because of the inducement, it made my body feel further along in the process of birth. I told Christian as a few hours passed that I felt I was at 8 cm. I felt like I was beginning to lose control. I now needed to lie down. I was starting to shake and my body was taking over.

The nurse came in and she wanted to check my progress. She told me again that I was at 3 cm. I couldn't believe it. This was awful pain, how could it only be 3 cm? I looked at the clock and it was around 10:30 p.m. or so. I remember thinking that I couldn't do this much longer. I was exhausted and I wanted to stop it all.

THE HEARTBREAK OF STILLBIRTH

Christian held my hand and rubbed my back, trying to offer me comfort. He was constantly praying over me and holding me. He was so broken. We both knew labor wasn't going to be the hardest part. After the nurse checked me, my friend Darby came up to me and whispered some words of hope to me. She was trying to convince me that I was almost finished and praying for me that I would feel God was near.

Soon after I lay back down, I told Christian to hold my hand and to call for the nurse. I began to push. I felt like I was going to throw up. They tried to get me to wait, but I couldn't stop. They called the doctor but there was no time.

I was ready to push and he was about to be born. Things were happening so fast in that room. It felt to me as if people were racing around, but we were sitting still. We were frozen in that moment holding onto one another and they were in fast forward like some kind of movie. We were grasping onto each other and knowing the proverbial car we were driving was about to wreck. He was coming and sadly I could feel those mother's emotions at the end of birth. I was excited that he was going to be on my chest in a few moments. I was going to meet my son.

Malachi Arrives

I actually felt joy that he was almost with us. I was excited to see him, to meet him, to hold him. I pushed a few times and he was delivered. The nurse was the one who delivered him. I think the resident came in right at the end. In my mind, it felt like at that point there were several nurses and residents coming in and out. I remember seeing nurses and doctors who I had never seen up until the moment I was pushing. Darby was out of the room waiting as we delivered him. She later told me that every nurse and doctor who left that room had been crying. Grief and sorrow for our son filled that room.

The Birth

The nurse placed him on my chest just as we had asked. He was so perfect. He looked just like his siblings. His eyes were closed. His mouth was slightly opened. His hands were together and placed perfectly upon his cheek. That is how he was born — those tiny hands upon his sweet face. He looked so peaceful. Our little boy.

I feel like the moment he was born I cried so loud that it was heard from here to heaven. My sorrow couldn't be contained. My heart was torn apart. He was here and only for a little while. He was so perfect, but he couldn't stay with us. He was going to have to leave us.

I am not sure how long I held him before Christian held him. But I remember how moved he was when he picked up his son. His eyes were filled with so much pain, like his heart had been ripped out. He just shook his head and cried as he held his son. Sobs came right from his heart into that room. His sorrow and tears were dropping right down on his little boy's body. There we were weeping and gazing at him. He was beautiful.

There is nothing that I can compare this to in my life, this type of pain and torment. I have always been aware that death was real. But it always seemed that death was far away, as if tragedy wasn't meant for us. Not that we were above it — it just felt like it wouldn't happen to our child.

It was so sad knowing that his siblings at home would never get to know him or even see him. We had decided that it would be too difficult for them to come to the hospital. We thought it would be best for them to see him through pictures. With everything that they had to try to understand in the next few days, we didn't want them to have more than they could handle. We already were going to have to explain what happens when a person dies, where they go, why their bodies are still here but their spirit is gone with Jesus, why there is a casket, and why their brother had to lay inside of it. It was too much for them. It was too much pain too fast. We decided this for their protection.

Even today, as I write this book, they ask me why they didn't get to hold him. We try to explain it all to them. The reality is that as their parents we had to make a very difficult choice. They can see him whenever they want in his pictures, but we understand that it is hard for them. They just want to hold their brother.

After we held Malachi for a long while our families came. It took a little while for people to arrive. Each person had a chance to hold him, and each person wept, completely grief-stricken. The scene was just heartbreaking.

For the first time, my sisters and I had all been pregnant together at the same time. We were thrilled that our kids would be born so close together, within months of each other. Today, I hold their sons, play with them, and adore them both. But each time I am with them, I know that my son is missing. As I watch their boys play, celebrate their birthdays, and hear stories about what they do and say, I wonder what Malachi would be doing. I wonder what he would love, what he would say that would make us all laugh, what he would do that would get himself into trouble. I am so thankful that my sisters have their sons with them. I am so grateful to have those boys in my life.

Everyone who came to the hospital looked at Malachi with such wonder and such love, knowing that this would be their only time to ever see him and embrace him. It is so devastating to watch the family and friends that you love hold your child and weep and watch each of them say good-bye and let their little nephew and grandchild go. We realized in those hours that although we would suffer the worst of this pain, our families were going to suffer and grieve alongside of us.

I'll just start to talk...I'm in this place where I think about leaving him a lot. I think about holding his little body and feeling like I am going to run with him outside the hospital and run away with him. I know that sounds crazy.

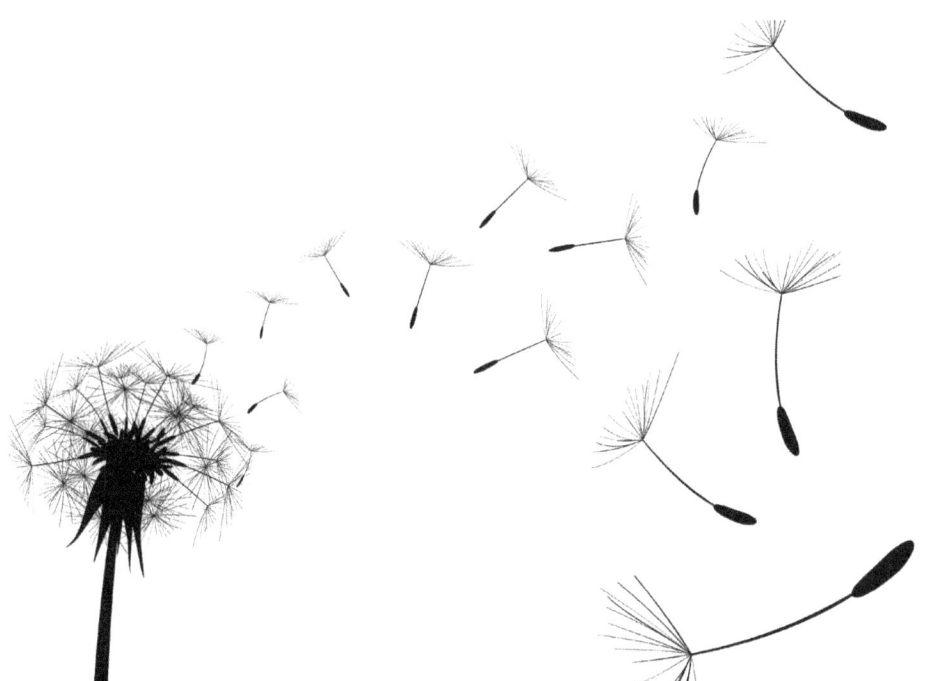

3

Leaving

If giving birth was hard, leaving Malachi at the hospital was harder still. Sometimes I feel like I am right there, holding him again in that hospital room. I couldn't let Malachi go. Christian had to come and talk to me and then take him from me. I feel so terrible even now because I know that I made Christian's journey in leaving our son that much more painful.

It was late in the very early hours of the morning. I was holding Malachi in the rocking chair, feeling the smooth rocking motion and trying to not fall asleep. At one point, I just wanted to stay and sleep with him on my chest. I would close my eyes for moments and then open them to the reality that he was dead. I would look down at him and see his little face and try to come up with ways that I could still keep him. Ways that I wouldn't have to leave him. Thinking of things that would enable me to take him home. My heart hadn't let his death set in…not yet.

Eventually Christian came over and told me that it was nearing the time that we should think about going. Our children would be awake soon. We had been gone for a full day and our kids had just been thrown into all this grief as well. They needed us to be home. We knew that this meant that we had to say good-bye. I remember telling Christian that I couldn't do it — I couldn't give him up — I didn't know how to let him go.

I sat there in that rocking chair sobbing. I told Christian that I wasn't going to be able to walk away. I couldn't leave him. I became distressed that we had to leave and I began to throw so many questions out in my distress. I kept saying, "Why didn't God save him?" "Why do we have to do this?" "We wanted him! We prayed for him!" Christian then told me the first words that brought me comfort since we found out Malachi had died. He said, "I don't see it this way. I see God giving us Malachi as an honor. God chose us to have Malachi because He trusted us with him."

Christian realized that God wasn't just taking a child from us. He realized God had given him to us. He wanted to believe in that moment that God was the author of life and He knew when Malachi was formed that his life would be short here. But God knew that we would seize him and take hold of the life that He had allowed us to have.

I will never forget that moment. Those words still ring inside my head. To this day, I feel that God gave us a gift that He trusted us to hold. In so many ways I cannot grasp how he has changed me and my family. I am just beginning to see all that God will do through our son Malachi.

Malachi isn't just another tragedy in this world. His life will forever hold the meaning of his name: "messenger of God," and "angel."

Saying Good-bye

After we said our final good-byes to Malachi, Christian laid him on the baby bed and covered him with a blanket as if Malachi were going to sleep. He left his face out of the blanket, and he looked so peaceful. Christian came over to me and told the nurses that we were ready to go.

Leaving

We were on our way out and I looked over at Malachi and started to freak out. I didn't want him to be alone on the cold table. That thought was tormenting. I had to keep telling myself that he wasn't in that baby bed — that he was with Jesus. But inside I was falling apart. Malachi was alone, and it was more than I could bear. I never said a word…I just cried.

The leaving process felt like it took forever. I felt like I had the chance to change my mind and go and get him. Part of me felt like asking them to hurry and get me down to my car as fast as possible so I could get away from the pain and never have to walk this road again. The other part of me just wanted to go back to the room and pick him up and rock him again.

Christian went to get the car, and I sat in the wheelchair exhausted and emotionally a wreck. The nurses kindly told us to call if we needed anything. Still the moment wasn't right for words and they knew that. They knew that nothing could be said and that leaving was torture. I got into the car and we began to drive away. We both just cried. I just kept asking Christian, "How can we leave him?" I said, "He is just up there on that bed all alone." There is nothing that can compare to the moment when you are forced to say good-bye — when you are left with nothing but a body and asked to leave. Although labor was so painful and more taxing than any other, leaving Malachi was the most difficult thing that I had ever had to endure. It didn't matter how much I wanted to go back or how much I wanted this to all change — he had died. I had to let his physical body go.

When we came home it was almost light and we knew that the kids would be awake soon. We went upstairs and we stood in the kids' rooms. We kissed them, covered them up, and gazed at them for a while. We felt so overwhelmed with emotions. We got into bed and we both took our Bibles. I felt in the moment that I got my Bible out because I had to, not because I wanted to hear from God. I needed to read something that would tell me God hadn't left me. I was exhausted but my heart wanted to know that He hadn't turned His back on me.

Why is this happening? Why is he gone? I just want to hold him a little longer—just a little. I want to sit there in that rocking chair and see him again.

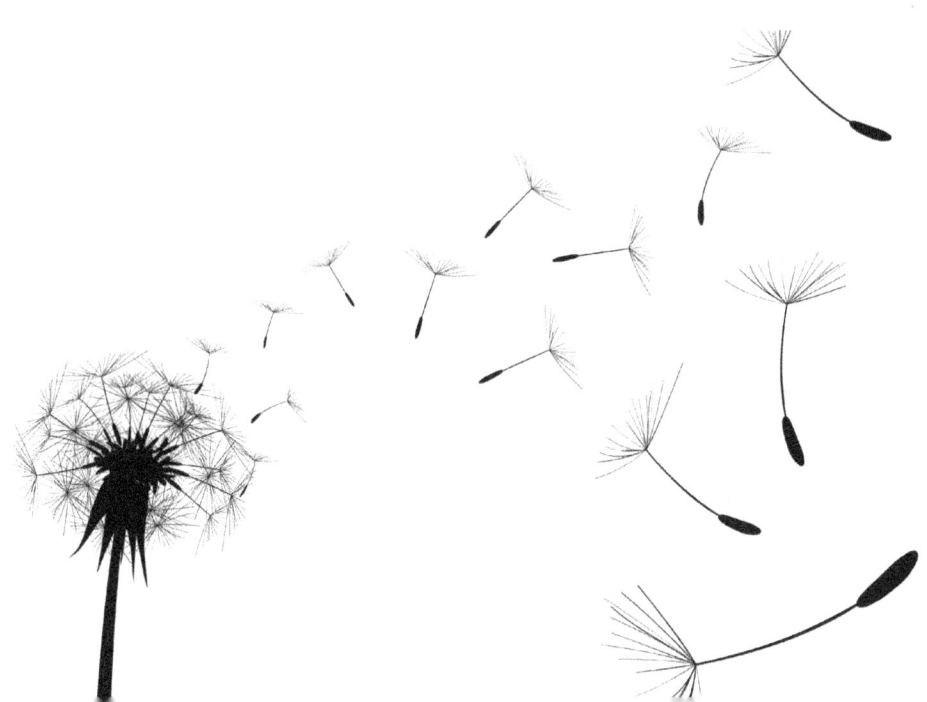

4

Back to Normal

The day after we delivered Malachi, we awoke to a house with kids that had many needs. They were emotional and so were we. We didn't know how to act and we couldn't, nor did we want to, hide our grief. They saw us break down and sob. They saw those who visited us come in crying and embrace us.

They were almost vacant in emotion. We expected this reaction. Since we were so visibly upset, I think they inwardly chose to put their emotions on hold. They definitely had outbursts and moments of true release, but during those first few days it just felt like a roller coaster. Their innocence was lost. Their knowledge about death was changed so quickly. They had all these plans for when their brother arrived — all these tasks they wanted to be able to do to help him. For example, we always have the kids buy something that they pick out for the new baby. They give this gift when the baby comes home, so that they can feel that they have a present to welcome him.

We hadn't purchased these gifts before we found out about Malachi's passing. So, the night before his funeral, we took them to the store so that they could buy presents for their brother. It was so painful to watch them pick out presents that they would have given to him if he had come home. It was just so beautiful to watch them look around the store trying to find the perfect gift that they wanted to give. They were so little, yet they wanted to give their brother a present that only they could give. It was amazing. Their hearts were so pure. This exciting present had turned into their final earthly gift for their brother. You could see how important it was for them to do this.

This special gift that has been a tradition to welcome a new family member had turned into them saying good-bye. The oldest one picked out socks and a basketball. The middle one picked out shoes and a football. The youngest one picked out pacifiers. They laid them on Malachi's coffin after the service. It was so heartfelt. They put them up there and they all just stood there looking at them. The funeral director told us he knew how important it was for the kids to give these gifts. He told us that after we left he would open the casket and place them inside where they belonged.

An Outpouring of Love

We received so many meals, flowers, cards, and baskets from so many people. Our children were able to see how much people loved us through this outpouring. They also received many toys and gifts from family and friends. People wanted to give them something to do and something new to take their minds off of their pain.

I am thankful for everyone who took the time to reach out to us. It was so comforting to hear the doorbell ring and get flowers or a basket of some sort or to open the mailbox and get cards and letters from people extending their comfort. The meals that came to us had been prepared with such love. We could tell that people had done more than the usual just to make it special for us.

Back to Normal

We had so much support and love, but I couldn't help feeling incredibly alone. My kids went about their day asking questions one minute and needing to cuddle or play the next, while I was there lying on the couch crying most of the day. I know it was good for them and they needed to see us grieve their brother. But it was difficult for me because I also didn't want to cause them any additional pain. Often, I would go to the bathroom and grab the hand towel, cover my face, and weep. I had to get it out. Between getting them dressed, making meals, and trying to keep up, I would find myself needing to let out the tears.

Death is so cruel. We had a baby that we could not bring home. And yet we were forced to follow the same guidelines as if we had him right there with us, recovering together from birth. I was limited in physical activity. I was supposed to rest and recover from going through birth. It felt like such a mockery. I wanted to be nursing my baby, but he wasn't there in my arms to enjoy that precious time with.

There is just this time that new parents are supposed to get with their little one. The baby is so new and they need so much attention, whether it's nursing, diaper changing, burping, rocking, or just kissing because they are so adorably wrinkly. When you deliver a stillborn baby, you don't get any of these things that you have been looking forward to, not to mention a lifetime of events that you will never get either.

You do not have all those reasons to wake up. Your reasons are all about grief. You don't sleep because you wake up sick with grief. I remember waking up each morning and as soon as I would open my eyes, I cried. It was as if I had to relive his death each morning. I awoke realizing that he had died and there wasn't anything I could do to bring him to life. I would just lie there and cry. Christian would wake up to me crying and he hadn't even opened his eyes yet!

That realization is a deep sick feeling right in the pit of your stomach. Your body needs to rest and recover, but your heart has just begun to grieve and you have to find a way to get up and make it through each day.

I tried to rest but all of my thoughts would be on letting him go. I would lie on the couch and then get up out of complete anger. Christian would say, "Mandy, you need to rest. Please go lie down and sleep." And my reply was often, "What for? There is no reason." He was desperate to get me to lie down and to sit still, but I refused over and over again. I was up and down the stairs, getting stuff for the kids, doing laundry, and cleaning. You name it, I was doing it. I was sore and in pain, but I didn't care.

When I had babies before, I would come home to kids and a house of chores to do, but it was drastically different coming home without Malachi. In the past there were so many reasons to stay down and rest — so many obvious reasons to recover from birth. This time I didn't see the purpose in resting. I had no baby to hold and nurse. I felt empty and lost. When you bring a baby home there is an acceptance of why the mother sits and rests. I almost felt guilty for resting. I would lie down and then tell Christian, "This is stupid. I do not want to lie here. Who cares if I don't recover?" I was so angry and hurt. I just wanted Malachi to be in my arms.

It didn't help that I am stubborn! But after some medical issues began to arise, Christian became worried and finally told me that I had to rest for a little each day. I tried but it wasn't easy. There was a moment when he told me something about them all needing me and that meant I needed to take care of myself. I knew that, and I wanted to be healthy for all of them too, but my pain was so deep that I just wanted to run in some way.

I read many books on stillbirth, grief, and losing a child. I would try to take small naps but every time I started to fall asleep I would get panicked and adrenaline would rush through me. I didn't want to keep waking up to my horrible reality. I just wanted everything to go back to when I was pregnant. Lying there with the house quiet meant me sobbing non-stop. There were so many times that literally my eyes and my head couldn't handle all the crying. I felt like my head was going to explode. My eyes were so puffy that sometimes it was painful. I didn't want to lie there and keep crying. It seemed easier to try to do something so I could get some kind of break in some way.

Fortunately Christian was there with me. He was able to take some time off from work and that was very helpful. We also had some vacation time that we had saved for when Malachi would have been born. The church was very gracious to us during this time and that was a huge blessing. They extended so much grace to us by being flexible and giving Christian freedom to return to work slowly. We know that not many people get this when they are grieving. There did come a day when he had to go back to work though. It felt so wrong. How were we supposed to just jump back into life and start where we left off? How was I going to take care of the kids when, emotionally, I couldn't take care of myself?

Jumping Back In

It was similar to when I had delivered our other children and Christian had to go back to work. I was in need of so much help physically but unwilling to actually have anyone help me. I was exhausted not only from labor, but from grief. My body was not anywhere near ready to accomplish all that I needed to do in one day. But at some point we had to jump in and take the plunge back into life.

One of the first nights that Christian had to work, our son had an emotional breakdown (we would soon become very familiar with these).

THE HEARTBREAK OF STILLBIRTH

I was barely holding on emotionally myself and I just needed to get the kids into bed so I could let it all out. They all were crying that Christian had gone to work. They were watching him leave and crying by the door and window. Then the "breakdown" occurred right before I got the kids into bed.

Our oldest son began to scream and cry — kicking the wall and saying, "I don't want Malachi to be in heaven with Jesus." He was angry. I sat there next to him and I told him that I wanted him here with us too. I said that I was sad that he wasn't here and that it was okay for him to be upset that Malachi wasn't here with us. He was starting to let it out. We knew it would come out; sometimes these things take time. I tried all I knew to get him to settle down so he could go to sleep, but nothing worked. I tried love and then I tried discipline. I just knew he was broken and it was all directed at his dad leaving for work. Finally in his broken voice he said, "I don't want Daddy to go to work and die."

It finally came out. He had fears and they were so real. He was confused and upset. I had no answers for him that would calm him. I knew that I couldn't promise that Daddy would come back. That would have been lying to him. All I could say were things like, "I think Daddy will be back, but if he does die then God will take care of us." "Bad things do happen sometimes but God always takes care of us." I was at a loss for words. I knew that he wanted me to say the exact thing that I shouldn't say. He wanted me to promise him that his dad wouldn't die — not just that night, but that he would be with us forever. He wanted me to give him security.

On another night our middle child out of nowhere told me, "Mom, when I get to heaven I am gonna run to Malachi." I couldn't hold back my tears. It was such a surprise to me that he would think to say this at four years old. It was so precious that in his little heart, he was having such powerful feelings. All by himself he was thinking that he would be so excited to see his little brother that he would have to run to him! It was so sad (and happy at the same time) for me that he was preparing to have this embrace with his little buddy and thinking about him and missing him.

This routine went on for sometime when Christian would leave for work in the morning too. The kids would each have their meltdowns and then we would try to start our day. It was extremely challenging to face each day, and I am not sure I always knew what to do or say. But they knew that we loved them and that we were going to walk with them through their pain. We weren't going to let go of them. Nothing could stop us from walking with them through this pain. Just like our Heavenly Father wasn't going to let go of us in our pain and grief.

The Little Things
I hated the idea that there was a "grieving time" and that all of my pain in some way had to come out in those first weeks. I hated that all of my tears were expected to happen in that allotted time or else I was considered some kind of therapy project. I knew that this would be more than coming home from the hospital and burying Malachi. At some point I had to let go of what everyone else thought. I had to let go of what was expected of me and allow my heart to keep grieving.

Slowly I learned that each day is a task within itself. Each day it is a choice to lay him down all over again and make myself embrace what God has for me that very day. This is never an easy task, and in the beginning it was almost impossible.

Getting up and just getting ready was difficult. Little things like getting the mail and seeing the baby flyers that I was receiving because I had been pregnant. It had my name on it, it was for me and for him, but we now had no use for these coupons and notices. He was gone.

I walked into the grocery store one day soon after he had died and the woman from the bakery who gives our kids cookies saw that I wasn't pregnant any longer and she said with such a happy face, "Oh! You had your baby!" My kids looked at me and their mouths fell open. They were still and quiet, waiting to see what I would say. I tried to gracefully say that he was stillborn and that now he is in heaven and we missed him but were holding on. Then I tried to change the topic so she wouldn't feel uncomfortable. She was quite wonderful and actually shared a story of loss that she had experienced. I felt badly for her. People don't usually know what to say and they just feel so badly for not knowing. But I knew it wasn't her fault. How could she have known?

Another time I was at a large store that carries everything from food to clothes and I had to pass the newborn section. I just looked and stared at it all. I saw pregnant women in there just browsing for their little one. I couldn't help but think, "Why Malachi?" I didn't want their babies to die, I just didn't want him to have died either.

On a different occasion, I was in a store shopping for a baby shower and I saw these adorable baby blue crocheted booties. They were so sweet and just the right size for a newborn. I held them and I wanted them for our boy. I would have bought them if he had been with us or if I had still been pregnant. I started to cry right there in that aisle. My eyes were filled with tears and I couldn't help myself. No one knew and if anyone saw me they probably thought I was crazy. They were the sweetest little shoes I have ever seen.

The tears really can happen anywhere — baby showers, grocery stores, the mall, even going for a walk — and suddenly your heart is thrown again into a sudden shock that your baby is gone. A few weeks after Malachi died, I needed to put away the maternity clothes and give back what I had borrowed from my family and friends. I couldn't fit into my regular clothes, and trying to find anything to wear was completely depressing. I needed to get these maternity clothes out of my closet and into storage. I kept telling Christian that I wanted him to give them away but we stored them anyway.

As I opened up my closet and began to put them away, my heart sank with each piece of clothing. I stood there in my closet and saw them hanging there and all I wanted to do was throw them out my window. I was so hurt and angry that these clothes were being taken away from me. It is a small window of time that a woman gets to be big and glow. I just wanted to be able to use them. I couldn't stand looking at them, but I also didn't want to get rid of them.

I saw the things that I had worn the week Malachi had died. I had to put away the very outfit that I had worn to the hospital. I had borrowed many clothes from my sisters and friends, and now I had to give these back. But the situation wasn't such that I was thankful to be on the other side of the journey having given birth and now enjoying having our son with us. I didn't get to enjoy the place where you look at the maternity clothes and you are so excited to be out of something that has a pouch sewn into it. (I mean really, what other time in life do women have extendable pouches on their stomachs?) And I didn't get to experience the joy of being able to see my toes again and tie my own shoes without help from someone else! That is a great place to be in after you deliver your baby. When you have a stillborn baby, all of these things are objects and emotions that you would run a marathon to get back. You covet the maternity clothes. You cry when you bend over and there is no baby stopping you from tying your shoes. It hits you like a speeding train.

As I put all of the clothes away, I cried. What else could I do?

THE HEARTBREAK OF STILLBIRTH

Christian came in and out of the room to just hold me. He kept telling me that he would do it or he would get someone else to do it. But there was just this part of me that needed to do this job. I felt as if someone would be taking a part of my memories of Malachi if they put these clothes away instead of me. That may sound like an exaggeration to some — but for each person it is different. Some may not feel this way and would love to have help. They may need someone else to put the clothes away for them, because it is too painful for them on their own. Personally, I needed to be the one who let these memories go.

Learning to Walk Again
At times, I felt that I didn't want to go on at all. Not that I wanted to end my life — I just didn't want to live it without Malachi. I know that seems impossible: you either want to live or you don't. However, I was in this place where I wanted to be here with Christian and the kids but I just couldn't bare the idea that I would be without Malachi. Still I feel these things, but as time goes on it is different. It is not less pain necessarily, just different pain.

I have realized my heart will never be the same as it was before we lost Malachi. I won't feel joy like I used to, or even pain for that matter. I am learning how to walk out each day. I don't think you can lose a child and then pick up where you left off. Not me anyway. I am figuring out how to ask God for help, how to love God in a new way, and how to believe His promises in the Bible. I can't just pick the ones that I like to hear, I have to believe them all or else He isn't who He says He is. I have to believe in my heart that He will not leave me and that He catches all my tears. I have to believe that death will not win in the end and that I will hold my son for eternity.

I think in making this choice I am allowing God to reach me in ways that He never has. That is difficult for me because I would have allowed Him to do this without Malachi dying, but He is going to use his death so that it brings good in our lives. Having Malachi has been a blessing that I cannot measure here on this earth. I feel so honored that he was given to us. I am so very thankful that God trusted us to have him in our family.

*It makes me feel so insecure. I now feel that there are no securities.
I knew there weren't really . . . but now it feels that even with my
prayers I cannot be safe from death or tragedies.
It feels so hopeless at times.*

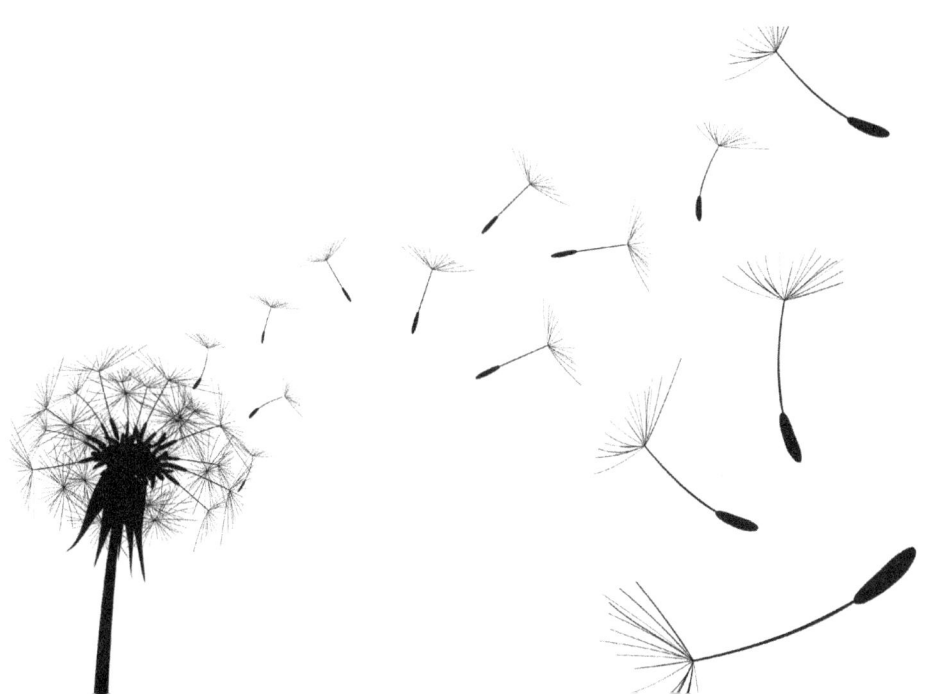

5

Surprised by Hope

I think the word expectant sums it all up. You begin to change everything in your life from the moment you find out you are pregnant. Every day is centered around your new little one. What you eat, how you sleep, what you wear — it all revolves around the little one inside you. As a woman you go about your day — throwing up, enduring pounding headaches, fighting leg cramps in the middle of the night, dealing with varicose veins and swollen body parts — and all the while you know it's all for a great reason. You have all these discomforts and you decide, "Who cares? This is so little for me to sacrifice for our baby." As you wake up in the morning, you possibly throw up (or feel like you are going to) and you think, "This is a good sign. Our baby is just growing and getting stronger each day." You watch your body change and expand. You begin to see the little one making his or her way to becoming bigger. You are approaching that fun stage where you no longer look like you have put on a few pounds, but you can actually wear maternity clothes.

This phase is so much fun. You get to rub your belly, and other people do as well — welcomed or not! But you can see this little one growing as fast as your excitement is. People start saying things like, "The baby is coming so fast! Before you know it, you will be holding this little one!" And of course, you can't wait. All the plans of your family become centered on this new arrival. Vacations, school, work, trips — you consider the whole list in the light of the baby's arrival. You clean like a mad woman. You try to paint and rearrange your universe before this little one hits the scene. You have a list of things to do and whether they are rational or not, you are determined to accomplish them. Then one awful day, it happens. Let's face it: your once exciting life filled with joy and wonder suddenly becomes a living nightmare.

It doesn't matter what you planned, how excited you are, or what you have changed or prepared. It doesn't matter how much you wanted this baby, or how excited your children are. It even feels like it doesn't matter how much you prayed. It isn't in your hands; truly it never was.

I honestly never saw this coming. Not once, but twice, we were handed this reality. On June 25, the year after Malachi died, we found out that our daughter Hope had died in utero, just as her brother had. The reality was harsher and seemed much more cruel when we lost her. Her arrival seemed all too perfect. After we lost Malachi, we had no idea what path we would take. We didn't know if we would go on to have more children, but we were overjoyed when we found out we were pregnant again. Her life seemed like the perfect surprise — the kind of present that you knew you wanted but could not imagine ever getting. It is like seeing a gift in some store that you would love, but realizing that mostly likely you are not going to get this extravagant gift. You think, "How would that ever happen?"

But it did! I was pregnant again, and we were so excited. The kids were just thrilled. I can still remember them jumping for joy on our bed. They were screaming and shouting. It was a celebration of her life, a birthday party for their sister — as it turned out, the only party they were ever to have for her. They still talk about the day they found out I was pregnant with her. They still talk about how excited and surprised they were. This memory is just tucked back into their hearts.

    This used to be difficult for me. I felt so sad that they remembered a moment full of such innocent joy, and one that would so quickly be replaced with complete sorrow. Now I am thankful for this memory in their hearts. I am thankful that Hope heard them cheering with joy over her. I am thankful that she was embraced by her siblings in such an exuberant way. It took time, close to two years, but I am so thankful for their memories of this day. I am, because I have realized it is special to my living children.

    It may be a challenge for me to remember seeing them so full of joy and laughter when more tragedy was to come in their lives. It may be difficult for me to recall that day and see so much excitement and sheer joy. I feel angry on their behalf. I feel burdened inside that I could not shield them from additional suffering. I often remember that day with thoughts like these: "If only we had known…we could have prepared them in some way. We could have protected them in some way, shielded them from a portion of the pain that would come in losing their sister." I know none of this is true. I realize we cannot protect them from death. And no matter what we could have come up with to say, the reality is their sister was going home. Looking back now, I would not change that moment. In that moment we were together. In that moment, Hope was with her siblings and they were with her. Her life, so short-lived in many people's eyes, has forever been placed within our hearts.

    After we made our announcement about Hope's arrival in our lives, our oldest son asked, "Is this baby going to die too?" We were, sadly, prepared for this question. We answered then, as we did every day I carried her, "We do not know if this baby will live or die, but we know that we love this baby and we are thankful for this baby." The kids prayed every day that she would not die. Sometimes they prayed this throughout the day. It was so pitiful to hear that prayer each day. But it was even more pitiful that their fears became reality, their innermost fear realized.

As you might expect, we had waited to tell them about her. We waited until I was thirteen weeks along in pregnancy. We had an ultrasound, and she looked great. So we told them about Hope, thinking we were in the clear. But honestly, in this life, one is never "in the clear." No matter what we said or when we said it, Hope's life was not ours to have here. I wish somehow I could have spared our children from another loss — from more pain, more disappointment, and more cruelty. I wish I could have spared them from the pain that comes with watching so many other cousins and children they know be able to have what has been taken from them, not once but twice, but I could not.

They were expectant. They were soaring high with the thought of having another living sibling, not one that would take the place of Malachi, of course. That would not be possible. But this was a sibling they would get to have here. A sibling with whom they could share all the kisses, the hugs, the play times, and the love that all start the first day they know of that baby. They were so excited to have her, and to lose her was just crushing for them. Knowing as a parent that I cannot take that pain away, or lessen their burden, is often a weight too immense for me to bear. Even to this day, I watch them pick out presents for other little ones in our lives and it breaks me every time. Seeing them so thrilled to choose a toy or clothes for someone's baby and to see their faces overcome with that sparkle and that joy. It is a selfless joy they carry. They cannot wait to give their gift. They want to surround that little one with their love.

The Worst Day of Our Lives…Revisited

I felt numb. The same midwife who had listened for Malachi's heartbeat and discovered that he had died, was now desperately trying to find Hope's heartbeat. Again, I lay there waiting. Waiting to hear Hope. But no heartbeat was to be found. I had been in the exam room for a while and Christian was in the waiting room with our kids. He popped his head in with a smile and a curious look. The midwife turned to him and said with great desperation, "Christian, we can't find a heartbeat!" For a brief moment, he couldn't believe her. Then as it hit him, his head fell down. He looked at me and said, "You are kidding me!" I just shook my head. I could see the anger on his face and hear it in his voice. Despair washed over him.

Christian standing in that doorway is a vivid picture of how we came to feel. He was half in and half out of the room. He was both in immediate despair and also needing to shut the door and play with the kids, not telling them there was a problem. What were we going to do? How were we supposed tell them again that their sibling had gone home? He waited for me to come out of the room. The midwife made arrangements for us to go to the hospital, but we had things to do before going. She offered to help us tell the children. We declined. I was crying and visibly upset when I exited the room. They began to ask questions and we just said, "We will talk to you in a minute. Let's go to the van."

When we got into the van, we had them all sit down and we turned to them and told them the devastating news. We told them that when Mommy was in there they could not find the baby's heartbeat. We explained to them that she had died. Samuel just screamed right away. His anger and hurt came right to the surface. He began to kick the chair and released his tears in anger. Elliot's little face became consumed with sorrow. He didn't cry, not just yet; he just was shocked and sat in his car seat with no words to say. Mathea repeated to us what we had just said, "The baby is dead." I know it sounds harsh and even blunt. However, she was two and a half. All things are blunt at that age. We talked for a while and explained how Mommy didn't know, and that we had no idea that Hope was sick. We told them if we had known, we would have sought help for her like we do for them when they are sick. We tried to explain that it is more difficult to know if babies are sick inside a mommy's belly. We told them we would have to go to the hospital soon and they would be babysat while we went. It was so sad to leave them when they were heartbroken. It felt so wrong. However, the simple fact was we couldn't be in two places at once.

When we arrived home from our appointment, Samuel went directly downstairs and put together a song on his guitar for the baby. He came up and played it for us before we left. It was just precious. He was trying to express his grief and his pain. It was evident this would be just the beginning for all of them.

Before we went to the hospital, we felt that we wanted to go to the church and pray for a miracle. We called our pastors and some close friends and asked them to gather around us and pray that the baby would be given life. We asked them to pray that when we got to the hospital, there would be a heartbeat and the baby could be saved. I am sure to most of you this sounds like a long shot. As a Christian, I believe that the same power that dwells in Christ was given to us when He died on the cross. That includes the power to pray for the sick to be healed and the dead to be raised. It is okay with me if you find this ludicrous. It is fine if you think this attempt was in vain. This was a road we had to take in our faith.

I don't remember a whole lot of what we said to each other on our way to church. It is mostly a blur. I do recall talking about what we wanted from the people who were praying for the baby. We didn't want a room of mourners; we wanted a room filled with faith on her behalf. We told the people that if she had died, there would be time for tears, but right now we needed to seek the Lord for her life. The friends who prayed with us were all so wonderful. Of course, there were tears in that room but the prayers they offered were so powerful. It was in that prayer session that God gave me her name. I vividly remember sitting down and getting this vision of her being wrapped in the womb. It was like a blanket that was see-through, being wrapped and wrapped around her body. I felt the Lord telling me that He was wrapping this little one with hope. It was a beautiful vision. I am so thankful He spoke to me in this way. It still remains in my heart, and it is a beautiful picture for me as her mother to know my baby was being wrapped in a love that I could never manufacture for her.

    After we prayed, we wanted to go to the hospital and have an ultrasound. As we were driving to the hospital, Christian and I talked. We weren't blind to the fact that the Lord may not give us our request for her life. I told Christian that if the baby had died and it was a girl, that I wanted to name her Hope. I felt the Lord had given me that name in prayer. He loved the name and immediately agreed.

    Sadly, we knew the process we would have to go through when we arrived at the hospital. We had just been through it less that one year before. Some of these memories are crystal clear. Some are in a dense fog. I don't remember doing paperwork. I don't even remember talking to many people. I just remember being escorted upstairs to this maternity wing that had pregnant women who looked as if they were bedridden for one reason or another. I vividly remember seeing one woman lying in her bed. She looked so hopeless. So sad. So alone. I am not sure why she was there and in my despair I thought, "At least your baby is still alive."

THE HEARTBREAK OF STILLBIRTH

Cold, I know. But I was on a floor with women whose babies were still living.

Waiting for God

We were taken to the very back room. Again, it was a delivery room. They wanted us to be taken away from all the rush of the day in the maternity ward. This was so kind of them, even though it seemed ironic where they placed us. We were in this delivery room waiting for an ultrasound for almost an hour. They were really busy. The nurse was more than kind and came in a few times to check on us. There wasn't anything she could do, but we could tell she felt very burdened for us. As we were waiting there, I remember we took in the surroundings of the room. Once again, this room was made for a live birth. The baby bed, the monitors, and the whole room was setting the stage for welcoming a little one. I began to have a panic attack. I stood up and told Christian, "I can't do this again. I can't be in here. I want to leave. I can't do this again."

There wasn't anything Christian could do for me. There was no remedy. He couldn't tell me that we could leave or come back later. We had to stay. We had to keep waiting. And while we waited, we strived to still have hope.

So we just sat in there and waited. We didn't even talk much. We just stared into space. I remember knowing Christian was really angry internally. I could see his disappointment toward God. He just was sitting there and I could tell he was drowning in feeling like God had failed him. But I had no words to encourage him. Looking back, I realize that waiting in that hospital room for the definitive ultrasound is when I first remember knowing I had nothing to offer Christian. The only thing we could both do was to wait. We had to wait and see if God had raised her from the grave.

I don't remember getting to the ultrasound room. When we got there before the technician arrived, we prayed once more for a miracle. We prayed that there would be a heartbeat — that somehow she would still be alive. Unfortunately, the technician wasn't as gentle and compassionate as the one we had with Malachi. She was actually kind of blunt and detached. For us, that made this horrible time even more difficult. She was clinical, and her attitude made my tears seem hollow. I could see Hope on the machine. I could tell there was no heartbeat. I could see that there was barely any fluid around her. I remember asking, "Is there a heartbeat?" I remember her saying in a very matter of fact tone, "Oh no." It was as if she was saying, "Of course not."

In a very clinical way she began pointing out that she was dead. She showed us where the heart was and that there was no heartbeat. She showed us how her fluid was low and described some potential problems that could have taken her life. Part of me didn't even want to hear the facts she was saying. The other part of me wanted to understand a reason why she had died. We didn't stop her from telling us these details. I look back now and see how that was an inappropriate time to give us those details. The overseeing doctor came in and confirmed her findings.

We had a little girl, but she had gone home.

I know it seems hard to believe, but I have no idea what happened after this. I think we went back to the room where we had waited to talk about her delivery. I am pretty sure this is where we went. I do remember deciding we would wait a day to deliver her. We decided this for our living kids. We wanted to be with them for a day and take some time to grieve with them.

This was a difficult choice. It was taxing enough waiting for the following day to deliver Malachi. With Hope, I walked around for another entire day and then some with her in my belly, knowing she was gone. My kids would still kiss my belly. They would come up and pat and rub my belly. It was just torture. We made this decision to wait so that we could give the kids a little more time to process all that had happened. We also needed some time to organize who would be taking care of our living kids for the next forty-eight hours.

The kids also wanted to buy gifts for Hope, so we went to a baby store. Walking around a baby store full of pregnant women, moms, dads, and grandparents picking out baby items, and knowing my family would never be able to, was one of the hardest things I have ever done. Our kids were so excited to find clothes and toys for her. It was so painful watching our kids get excited about what they had chosen for their sister, knowing that she wasn't going to get to keep those things. It was important to them that they had something to give her. We couldn't take this away from them. Even though this was so difficult, it was the right thing for us to allow them to do.

I have this vivid memory of being in line and waiting to pay. My eyes were puffy and swollen from crying. Christian and I looked worn through and through. I recall standing there, feeling so very exhausted. I just wanted to crawl into a corner and deny my reality. Why wasn't I the woman in front of me who was buying a car seat? Why wasn't she me? Why was her child still living? Why did my family have to face death again?

We arrived home and the next thing I remember was my dad coming over. He came to check in and see how we were holding up. I remember my dad asking me if my daughter Mathea felt warm. I felt her and sure enough, she was warm. I took her temperature and she had a fever.

This felt totally ridiculous! Why in this critical state in our lives did my daughter have to have a fever? Of course, I couldn't wait until she felt better to deliver Hope. It had to happen the next day. Putting off her delivery wasn't an option. So, we had to leave Mathea and let other people care for her. If you know me at all (or can tell through this book) I want to be "there" for our kids. As any parent desires to be, I want to be available for them, especially when they are sick or hurting. Mathea getting sick just felt like God had allowed more pain and struggle for us in a time when it seemed we could not handle anything else.

Of course, our families and friends took amazing care of her. She wasn't crying or asking for us. She was in good hands. We had a rotation of care for our kids between family and friends. Knowing that this care was in place made leaving in the morning a little bit easier for me. Knowing that any one of them would do anything for our kids at a moment's notice set our minds at ease.

It was very early in the morning when we left for the hospital. Because we had a scheduled time to be at the hospital, the kids had to say good-bye to Hope the evening prior to her delivery. We were getting them ready for bed, they each took turns kissing my belly, rubbing my belly, resting on my belly, and talking to her. They told her how much they would miss her and how much they loved her. This was both beautiful and heart wrenching — to watch your living children say good-bye through tears to a sister they would never have the chance to see (other than in pictures) or hold or play with.

We had decided as we did with Malachi that it would not be beneficial for the kids to come into the hospital. I couldn't imagine waking up our two year old who was sick to come in. Allowing the boys to come to the hospital and leaving her out seemed damaging. For those of you who have let your kids come in after delivery or know someone who has, I'm not saying that's wrong. I wonder all the time if it would have been beneficial for them. Each of our children have expressed how they wish we would have allowed them to come and hold their siblings. But you don't have days to make this kind of choice. It is a decision you make when you have no resources and cannot think straight. For our kids I still think we made the right call. My point is that you need to find a way forward that will give you peace, knowing that God is leading you to what is best for your family.

We took tons of pictures so they could see her up close. We took many pictures of her, which today I am so thankful for — pictures of her being snuggled by us, of her hands and feet, and ones with her hat on. They "oohed" and "aahed" at her when we showed them. They laughed and smiled. They also had questions about her. We did our best to make these times of looking at her pictures times where they could ask us anything. It was meant to be a safe time for them to wonder and be honest with how they felt.

Leaving Empty Handed…Again
As we arrived at the hospital, the emotions I was experiencing were all over the map. You walk in and you are required to check in at the front desk. It is just so sad. It is the first person you come in contact with and you say, "I am here to be induced." They ask you a few questions (you can see the confusion on their faces as they scan the schedule for you) and eventually you are forced to say, "Yes, we just found out our baby died." One would think they would have some kind of system for this and know you are coming to avoid this painful discussion. My "normal" self would feel badly for the receptionist in that situation, but I didn't.

We proceeded to the delivery floor. This time, it was packed with women delivering. Babies were crying everywhere, the whole floor was "expectant," and there we were on the other end of the universe. We were placed in the same room where we delivered Malachi. It is the last room on the floor toward the back of the delivery ward. We had a feeling we would be in the same room. We had talked about this the day prior to delivery so it didn't really come as a surprise. However, it did make it very difficult for us. On the one hand it was special. On the other hand it seemed like torture. There wasn't another room left. Asking to be moved wasn't an option.

I vividly remember hearing the woman next door laboring. I felt like I was in some awful horror movie. I knew soon she would be holding her living baby and I would be hearing newborn cries. I felt sick. The whole idea that I was about to deliver my baby who was dead, while everyone else on the floor was delivering living babies, was too much to bear. I couldn't stop reality. I couldn't change what was going on. I was stuck knowing babies were being born and families were filled with joy. I remember my sisters coming in to be with us while I labored. My older sister wanted to go next door and tell the woman to "shut up." Ha! I thought it was funny. In times like these, sometimes humor is all you have to keep you sane. I didn't want the woman's joy to be taken away. Her day was special. Of course, she deserved to be totally thrilled and have her experience of delivery filled with excitement and happiness. It was just a complete challenge (to put it lightly) to listen to everyone giving birth and the clamor around the halls filled with laughter and little sweet newborn cries.

Soon the nurse came in and began the registration process. She began to tell us what would take place. We both just stopped her and said, "Sadly, we just did this almost a year ago. We know what lies ahead." She was apologetic towards our losses. She asked us what we wanted and then told me I needed an IV, to which I objected. I asked her to call the doctor and make sure it was necessary. I have no idea if she did or not; I genuinely can't remember.

THE HEARTBREAK OF STILLBIRTH

I think she just thought I was crazy. I told her I didn't want any medications. I told her I wouldn't be getting an epidural. She seemed surprised. Then I informed her that I had never had one in any previous delivery and didn't want this time to be the first time. She understood. However, she also explained that the option was there for me if I changed my mind.

Looking back, it would have been a great time to have an epidural. I mean, I was under so much stress. It would have been the perfect time to allow my body to have a break of some sort. But I am stubborn. Unfortunately stubborn. Sometimes in life stubbornness is wonderful. In this situation, it would have been helpful for me to look at the other side.

Instead, I was induced without an epidural. I can't remember the name of that horrid medication. It wasn't Pitocin. It was some other awful medication. It just made my body ache worse and worse like a slow torture. I have gone through natural childbirth and this medication just seemed to add more pain to the labor.

The process was much like it was when I delivered Malachi. The medicine was given every three hours until delivery. Toward the end of labor I began to feel as if I was losing my mind. I was exhausted. I was grieving. I wanted labor to end but knew that would mean beginning the process of letting our daughter go.

I know I said it before about Malachi, but normally you are supposed to be able to endure the pain of labor because you know that the joy of holding your new baby is just around the corner. With death though, the complete opposite is true. The only thing waiting for me after the pain of labor was the pain of letting her go. There was nothing good to look forward to.

My sisters stayed with us until I was ready to push. It is actually slightly humorous how they left. We told them that we wanted to be alone when she arrived. So as soon as I said, "I need to push," they ran out of the room so fast that honestly I only remember seeing the curtain rustling back and forth. They left so fast I never even saw them leave! Looking back it is humorous. Of course, in the moment I wasn't laughing.

I felt so sick and nauseated, but at the same time I knew I had to push. The nurse called the doctor. She knew the baby would come before he arrived. I gave my final push and there she was. So beautiful. The nurse commented on how sweet Hope was. She kept saying things like, "Oh, look at her little hands." It was just such a sweet way to receive Hope. She didn't treat Hope like she was dead. She treated her in such a special way. Most nurses and doctors are somber and don't comment on the beauty of your child. But she took the time and let us know how special Hope was. I was, and am, very grateful for this.

She laid her upon my chest and Christian and I just cried. We held her still body and wept a constant flow of tears. We would be crying and at the same time talking about all her amazing features, like how she looked so much like Mathea. Her mouth looked just like Mathea's mouth when she sleeps. She had chubby arms and legs. Her hands looked like Samuel's hands — wide little hands. Her hair was so sweet. It was really dark hair and there was this tuft on top that had a little wave to it. There is so much more I could say about what she looked like and how precious she was, but all of it wouldn't come close to fully describing the treasure that she was, and is, to us.

We took turns holding her. She was weighed and dressed. Then, slowly, our families came in and held her. They all took turns snuggling their niece and granddaughter. They all took turns saying good-bye. There are so many emotions to face. You are so proud to show off you newly born baby. But there was also so much sorrow and pain.

THE HEARTBREAK OF STILLBIRTH

When everyone finally left, we spent a long time holding her and loving on her. I didn't even want to get a shower because I knew I could always shower…but my time with Hope was limited. It doesn't matter how much time you spend. There is never enough time with someone you have to let go. At some point the nurses said to us, "Let us know when you are ready, and we can take her." I remember thinking, *So if I never tell you we are "ready," does that mean we can take her home?* I know that probably sounds ludicrous to you, but that's exactly how I felt.

The decisions you are forced to make match no others you have ever made before. We stayed with her for many hours. Then we began to talk about when we would leave. To even begin to give details about this process is futile. I mean, there are no words that can even come close to describing how one makes this choice. It is one that you always wonder about. Should you have stayed longer? How would you feel if you had? Would more time have been enough time? It is a process that is just laborious. The truth is, no matter how much time you take, it will never be enough.

Finally, we began to pack up our things. Because the maternity floor was so busy, the new change of nurses wasn't quite up to speed with us. They knew we were leaving, but everything seemed a little chaotic. I didn't want to ride in a wheelchair down to the car this time, so we didn't need to wait for a nurse to escort us out. Once you decide to go, it is almost like you have to put your heart on a deserted island. You leave a piece of who you are and you know you will not see it again until you go home to heaven. There is no going back.

We placed her in her baby bed. She was all bundled up in her little hat and sweet outfit. I kept adjusting the clothing on her. I just didn't know how to leave her. We kissed her and told her how much we would miss her.

Then, we left.

I looked back at her and again, I just couldn't believe I was leaving one of my children. She was going to be alone. She was just lying there by herself. We walked out of the room and down the hallway just clinging to one another and crying. We walked out of the hospital with our arms and our hearts completely empty.

Again.

*I cannot stop freaking out. It is a very lonely, desperate feeling.
I'll be watching my kids play and then it hits me and
I feel totally taken over....
I know I am depressed and I am just waiting for help to come.*

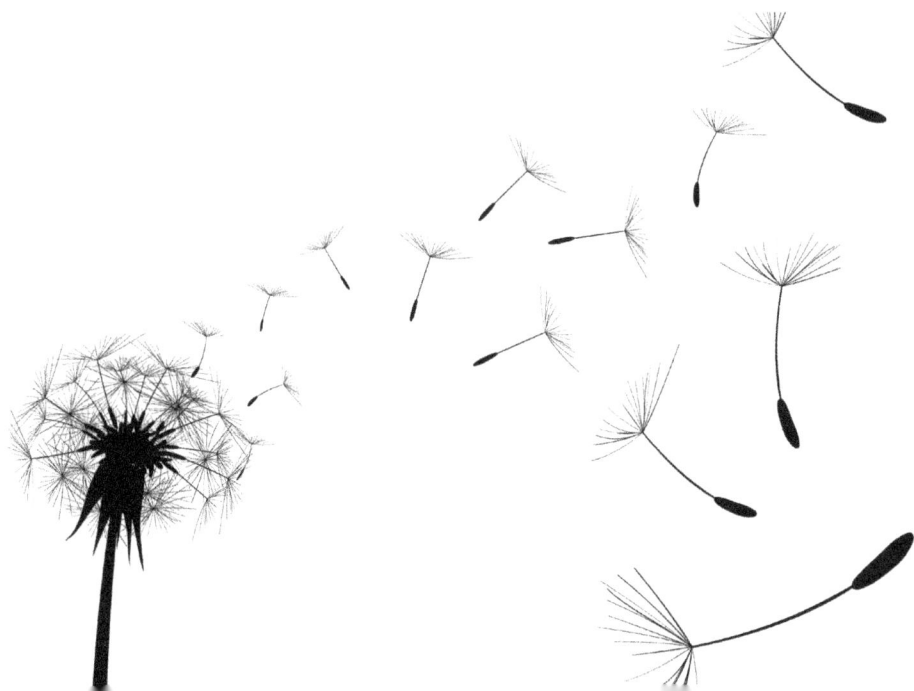

6

My Battle with Mental Anguish

A few months after we lost Hope, I started to go downhill emotionally. I know that sounds like I'm just stating the obvious. But it was much more than just mourning — which alone was already too great a burden to bear.

It was a year after Malachi died that we lost Hope. Actually, it was eleven months almost exactly. I began to become deeply depressed. At the same time, I was also struggling with extreme anxiety. I did not want to shower. I did not care if it had been three days, I just kept wearing the same clothes. Oftentimes, I would not even remember to brush my teeth. I didn't brush my hair or put on make-up. I wore huge sweatshirts and baggy jeans. Not that there is anything wrong with those clothes, but when you wear them three days in a row and then put them back on as soon as they are washed, there is something wrong with that.

I took care of my kids. I made them meals, did their wash, and took care of them completely. But I did not care about myself at all. I kept up with the housework, but not how I used to keep it. Instead of going the extra mile, I just did the bare necessities. I felt so much guilt. And the guilt did not help with the intense depression and anxiety.

THE HEARTBREAK OF STILLBIRTH

I would stay up late at night. I slept well when I was able to fall asleep (which is not the case for some people). Often, I would just stay awake watching TV or beading (making jewelry), or reading literature on the Internet about stillbirth. I was getting sleep, but I was all over the map. I wasn't getting the healthy six to eight hours of continual sleep one should get.

Suddenly, it all came crashing down. I had been through tons of testing and blood work because we had been led to believe that there was some hope for finding an answer as to why Malachi and Hope had died. It was a long shot, but it was all we had left. We thought this testing would be our answer to what our future would hold. We had put our decision (about possibly trying again) aside, and told one another we would wait until the results came back. Then, we would hopefully have the information we needed and wanted. We hoped this information would allow us to know clearly if it would be wise to "try again."

The doctor called and gave us the results. They were not in our favor. I remember that evening so clearly. I was making dinner and Christian was not yet home. I was crying on the phone with the OB. I apologized again and again for crying and rambling on. I think he talked to me for well over a half hour. He was filled with compassion. He knew how much we were counting on this test to give us some answers about our grief and our future.

I was cooking when Christian arrived home from work. He could see I was upset and I just shook my head. He knew what I meant. We had been expecting this call and he knew by my face that everything had come crashing down. I was so upset that we went into our powder room, sat on our bathroom floor, and I just sobbed. I kept telling Christian, "I think I am having a panic attack." My chest was tight, I could not breathe, and I felt numb in my legs. It was awful. It was just terrible.

All of my emotions about losing Malachi and Hope were slammed into my face. All of my hopes that maybe we would have an answer were lost in one phone call. Our dreams of possibly trying again, even though it sounded crazy to even think of it after what we had been through, came to a screeching halt.

We had been hoping the doctor would call with some kind of answer. As I've mentioned, there had been talk of a minor clotting issue. That would have been a simple answer for us: some kind of explanation to why we lost our children. I guess in a way that would have given a reason. Most people who lose a child through stillbirth know why the baby died: the cord was wrapped around the neck, placental abruption, a congenital malformation. These reasons don't lessen the pain. These reasons just give you a place for your heart to settle. It's something tangible you can blame. It doesn't mean having an answer makes your grieving easier. It just means you know why.

When the doctor called that evening, he explained that everything came back normal. Most of the time in life, that is a good answer! However, in our case it meant we would never know why our son and daughter had died. What we wanted was something to blame. Something to make sense.

This information (or the lack of it) stripped away all comfort. An answer meant I could do something if we decided to move forward and have more children. An answer meant our living children would have information they may need later in their lives.

I felt like God had taken everything. Because the doctor had found no reason, it meant I truly had no control. Without something to stand on, it meant God had to be in control. If I am to be totally honest, that wasn't what I wanted.

I wanted a say. I wanted the doctor to come up with a plan. I wanted to call the shots about our future and the future of our kids. This call made me feel like the only candle burning had finally been snuffed out.

After the news came, my emotions snowballed — from terrible to nightmarish. Now I was grieving and dealing with panic and anxiety. I became obsessed with a variety of things. I began to have panic attacks everywhere — at the grocery store, outside in the yard, and in my house. I began to be anxious in large settings. I would feel strange about a person at the park and feel cautious about their actions. The anxiety seemed understandable and tangible. It also seemed to make sense — even though it was frequent. With all that we were going through, it made sense I would have these emotions. These racing thoughts didn't seem strange to me in the beginning because I had lost two children. My fear, depression, and anxiety seemed understandable. I had experienced my worst fear not just once, but twice. Now it seemed that any bad thought that came into my mind had the possibility of actually happening.

I had people praying for me around the clock. I also met with my pastors on a regular basis. I hung scripture on my refrigerator and increased my Bible reading. I felt like it was a spiritual battle that I had to win. I felt I had to stand against the enemy and fight. I felt that the enemy was bringing more torture and using the anxiety to cause more pain and suffering. On some level, I am sure this was true. The enemy uses all opportunities to bring about more pain and wreak havoc. However, at this point, it was the chemicals in my body. I was totally depleted. Nothing was in balance any longer. My weary body was fighting back, but it had no clue how to do it and everything just plummeted.

As all of this escalated, my anxiety began to include paranoia. Fortunately, I was not clinically paranoid. I still knew the thoughts were irrational, and that is what separated me from true paranoia. Despite how difficult it is to share this, I chose to disclose some of this struggle about paranoia with you so those of you who are grieving, or know someone who is, can watch for these signs. Mostly, I share this so you can see how the death of a loved one is able to bring so many levels of pain. I hope this opens a door of understanding for yourself and compassion for others.

    I started to feel like people were after me and my family. Now, there is one difference apparently from truly being paranoid and having paranoid thoughts and emotions. The difference is that I knew these thoughts were paranoid thoughts and was able to recognize they were unrealistic; however, I was still not able to escape them. The thoughts would come and flood me even when I was not dwelling on someone or something around me. I was wrapped totally in fear. At this point it was a huge accomplishment for me if I went to the grocery store. It would take so much inner strength to allow myself and the kids to just go to the store. If anything was slightly off from the normal trip, I would come home a mess. I would go off away from the kids and call Christian or my sisters or pastor and just cry and ask for prayer. It would throw me off the whole day. I would have racing thoughts about what could happen. I knew they were just thoughts that were torturing me, but I could not escape them. No matter how hard I tried to pray or talk myself down, the emotions were right at the forefront. I felt like a prisoner.

    From there it progressed even further. Over time, the anxiety and the paranoia increased. The places that I felt "safe" became fewer and fewer. Instead of being able to go to the store, or take my kids to play in the creek, I just wanted to stay home. I would not go anywhere except for my sisters' houses and church. I did not feel safe anywhere. I felt that wherever I went, people were going to stalk me or take my kids. I knew it was not true. I knew it was totally irrational but I could not stop the feelings. It was torture. I hated having the thoughts, but I could not stop them. They swirled around my mind and consumed me. It was like my mind would get stuck on a track that just wheeled around and around.

I asked for prayer, read my Bible, got counsel, talked to people who also had felt this way before, but nothing helped. I would call Christian several times each day — often in tears. I just wanted him to come home. I felt safe if he was home. I would look out our window when the kids could not see me to see if anyone was outside. I just did not feel safe anymore. Eventually, the panic would come even without an event to provoke the thoughts or emotions. The chemicals were just soaring sky high through me and they were unrelenting.

At the height of these emotions our family was asked to go out to dinner with my extended family. I did not want to go, but I went for the kids because I knew it was not healthy to keep them at home. At the restaurant I began to think that people were looking at me strangely. My mind was racing and I could not even eat. I thought I was going to throw up. I just wanted to run out of the restaurant. Fight or flight was in full effect. I could feel the panic racing through my body. I was aware that these were just thoughts, and it wasn't something that was really happening, but I could not stop them. It was consuming.

We called our pastors and one of them came over later that night after our kids were asleep. He shared some challenges from his life that the Lord had brought him through. He prayed for me and spent a long time counseling us. We knew at this point that I needed to see a professional therapist and possibly a psychiatrist as well. Basically, I needed therapy and someone who could assess the issues and treat me accordingly. Of course, knowing that I needed this type of treatment just furthered my feelings that I was a terrible person. I felt that I was an awful wife and mother. I felt like I had failed my family. I felt that I had failed God.

My Battle with The Medication Stigma

I did not want to go to a therapist because I knew that she would want me to go on medication and I was terrified of that. But I went anyway. I had Christian and one of my pastors go with me. The therapist is a Christian and she was so gentle and loving. She did not make me feel like I was crazy. In fact, she assured me that I was in touch with reality. She also knew that medication would assist me in my mental and physical recovery.

I was wrecked inside about taking the medication. It may sound ridiculous and might be hard to understand why I would resist taking something that could help me. The thing is, I simply am not a medicine girl. For some reason, my body is sensitive to medications. I get nauseated at the drop of a hat with most medications. I cannot even tolerate over-the-counter sinus medications. I know, I sound like a wimp.

I know that medications serve their purpose and keep many people alive on a daily basis. I see the need for medicine, and I fully support the use of them when necessary. But that was just it — I was not in "need" of them to sustain my life. It made me feel so defeated. It felt in my heart as if I had not done what God needed me to do. I felt that by taking the medication, in some way I had failed God. I felt that I must have not prayed hard enough or applied scripture to my mind. I felt that I had lost a battle that I had tried in so many ways to win. I was not ill. I did not have a disease. So why take medication?

The therapist put the matter in simple terms for me. She said, "This is up to you. You do not have to take them, but you have fought so long and so hard and it sounds like your body just needs to have a break." She reassured me that it was my choice to make. She said she would be there to counsel me regardless of my choice. She also told me that I did not have to be on them forever. She explained to me I could go on them for a season and then go off of them when I felt it was time. I decided to go the medication route. After this meeting she referred me to a Christian psychiatrist.

I now understood that my problem was not just spiritual. It was chemical. My body needed to reboot. I needed to go on the medication and give my body the break that it so desperately needed. I could not manufacture any chemicals that I needed, so I had to allow the medicine to aid my body. I had tried vitamins and herbs but they did not help me. Maybe it has helped some of you and, if so, that is wonderful. Maybe if I had started them earlier, then they would have worked. For me, they just did not do the job.

The psychiatrist was helpful, but it was a difficult visit. I had to answer tons of questions so she could assess my mental health. It was challenging to sit there in that office. I felt ashamed and embarrassed. I felt that at any moment she would tell me that I was unstable and I could not be with my family and she would "admit" me. I was so afraid that I was going to be torn away from my family. Perhaps it's possible for you to see that under all of this fear, panic, and paranoia I was afraid of losing what was dearest to me. I had already lost two of my children. I did not want to lose again. That fear for me was real and justified, not simply based in my anxiety. Losing was a reality for me. It shook me again and again. It was not a false feeling that a therapist, a counselor, a pastor, or even medication could subdue. I had experienced this two times and I was terrified that it would be my reality again with my living children.

Christian and I talked again and again about the medication. We talked about how it may help. We discussed the possibility that I would have to try more than one medication to find the right match for my body. We discussed how it could be just temporary. I kept thinking if I went on medication, I would remain on it for the rest of my life, and that scared me. We talked about how I would feel about myself if anyone knew I was on medication. I mean, my husband is a pastor! His ministering wife is on antidepressants? Somehow that made me feel even more guilt.

Don't get me wrong. It's not as if I thought people in our church looked at me and saw perfection. That was not at all the case. There just seems to me to be bad feelings associated with antidepressants in the church "at large." I was afraid that if people found out I needed medication for anxiety and depression, they might think I wasn't following God closely enough, or that I was not receiving the joy and goodness God gives to His people. There was just so much there, so many deep thoughts about how I viewed myself and so many thoughts about how I felt people would view me and judge my heart. I felt like a failure. I was certain others would feel the same way about me.

I will never forget when I decided to take the medication. I was in church and I had some paranoid thoughts about someone who was at the church. I am not talking about discernment; I have that gift and it is strong in me. Having this gift also made the paranoia difficult to sift through at times. Was I discerning a dangerous person? Or was I just having paranoid thoughts? The line became foggy. I came to Christian in tears. I was worried about this person and I could not shake my emotions surrounding my thoughts about this person. I knew then that one of my last places of safety had been stripped away. All I had now was my sisters' houses. I knew in that moment that it did not matter if I wanted to start the medication or not. I had to do it for my family. I had to allow the Lord to start with me there.

It all came down to doing it for the kids. I should have wanted to do this for myself — for my own peace — but I just wasn't there yet emotionally. I wanted to be able to go places with my children and not be consumed with panic and paranoia. Even though I did not show it to them while we were out, I did not want to feel that way while we were out. I wanted to be able to discern again, to use sound judgment rather than being motivated by fear and anxiety.

God gave me so much grace through starting medication. I was able to go on one type of medicine, and it worked very well with my body and I have had good results. I was very adamant that I did not want to go on anything that would be addictive in any form. For me, I wanted to know I could go off the medicine and not have my body go into shock or be addicted in any way. So I started one of the mildest medications and, thankfully, it worked. Success with the first medication was a complete answer to prayer.

I have been on the medication for a good while now and I am so happy that I started it. I can assess situations and people's actions. When anxious or paranoid thoughts do come, they no longer consume mer. I can step out of the rising emotions, and I am able to judge with clarity what the situation may need at that time. It is such a freeing way to live. Once you have experienced the absolute depletion of these chemicals and then have them return, you feel free again, even though your pain is still present and your situation has not changed. You are no longer are a prisoner in your mind. If you have been here, you know what I mean.

As you can see, this decision was difficult for me. I know that is seems irrational, but it was truly an enormous challenge. Some people can see the signs and catch themselves before they are so depleted. I, on the other hand, waited too long before seeking help. The good news is that "we know that in all things God works for the good of those who love him" (Romans 8:28). I am hoping that He may be using all I went through to guide you now. The only advice I can offer is to seek professional help. Get the counsel and help you need. Be honest. Know you are very brave for acknowledging what you are going through. God is able to use even this destitute place to bring life.

True Help
It is painful for friends and family members to watch a loved one suffer. I know it was hard for those who love me the most to go through all of this with me, but their respect for me was a true blessing. My family members thought it would be best for me to go on antidepressants, but they also knew I had to come to that conclusion on my own.

What my family members did so well was to love me where I was and not force their ideas or wishes on me. I was in the deepest, darkest grief and they walked with me. Walking along side someone means holding them up. Think of the story in Exodus 17 (verses 8-15) where Aaron and Hur held up Moses's arms when he could no longer raise his hands when fighting the Amalekites. Aaron and Hur came alongside Moses and stood with him. He no longer had the strength in his own body to raise his hands (v.12). Aaron and Hur placed a rock for Moses to sit on and each of them held his hands up during the battle. As long as Moses's hands were raised, the Israelites were winning the battle. If his hands were lowered, they began to lose. This is such a strong representation of what I needed as I was suffering.

My friends and family could not take me out of the battle, and they could not overcome my enemies for me. Notice that Aaron and Hur did not try to convince Moses that he should just give in and rest his weary body. They did not tell him that the battle was too great. They did not try to deter him from the battle that was set before him. They knew that the battle had to be fought. So they did what they were able to do: they held him up.

I believe that what Aaron and Hur did for Moses is what my

loved ones did for me when I was suffering. I hope everyone who grieves has such support — the support of people coming alongside, providing a place to rest. We need others to hold us up during the battle when we no longer have the strength to do so ourselves.

The flowers are all dying.
For some reason this is hard for me.
I don't expect any more to come or anyone to send them.
I just don't want these to die.

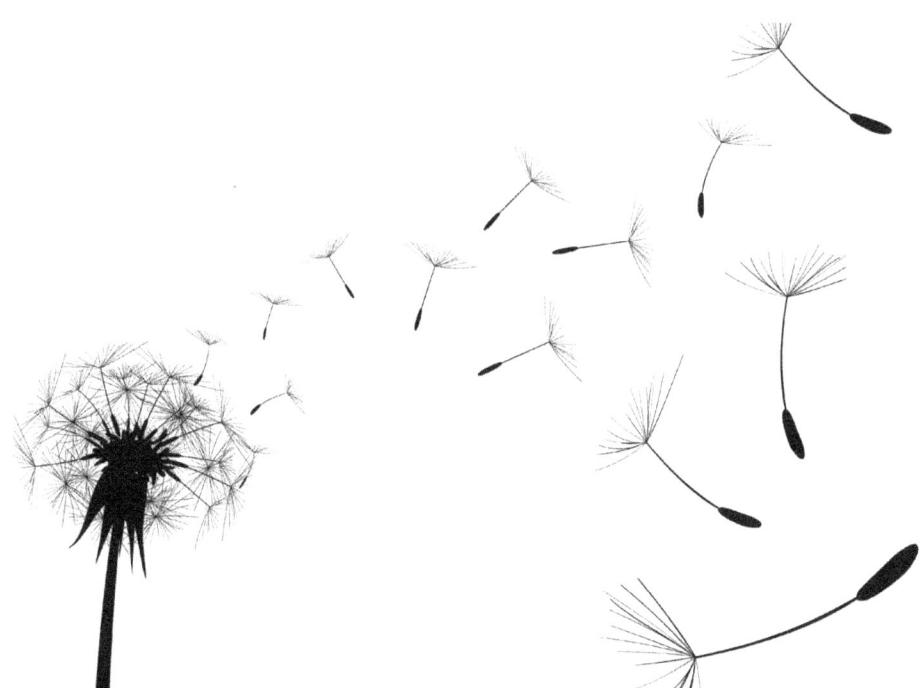

7

Freedom to Grieve

The reality is that death wasn't meant for us to grasp. We in our perfect beings weren't created to know death. It was sin that introduced that concept. Death is a temporary suffering "they" say. To a parent who has lost a child, that means nothing. It sounds good to say to someone who has lost someone close to them, "Your loved one is in heaven." Or, "They aren't suffering anymore." While those sentiments are true, they don't take pain away, or even do much to lessen it. What I mean is this: of course our loved one is happy in heaven. We are the ones stuck with the pain, guilt, and torment of their absence. Sure it all makes sense. They are where they want to be — with Jesus. But that doesn't make it any easier for me here. I am the mother left with her heart crushed. I am the one who doesn't get to hear the first cry, see the first breath, hold that little hand, and feel those pruned fingers clench mine. I am not a fool here. I know that Malachi and Hope don't want to return to this earth. But, oh, how my heart longs to embrace each of them once again.

God's Way for Me
Sometime after we lost our daughter Hope, I arrived at the place where

THE HEARTBREAK OF STILLBIRTH

I decided to stop searching for a way to "move on," and my grief began to make sense. Society wants you to move on and get through your grief. I feel that the Lord showed me I didn't (don't) have to grieve in this manner. I wasn't created to understand death and grief, and neither were you. The Lord created us to know and have life. He hates death so much that He put an end to our suffering through the sacrifice of His only Son. So instead of trying to swim through this ocean of grief and sorrow to find the other side, I decided to just sit down. Sound ridiculous? Why would I want to just sit in my sorrow and not try to search for a way out? Who enjoys sitting in agony?

This idea felt like the proverbial light bulb going on, like someone hit the switch and there finally was understanding. That moment for me was the moment of acceptance. I had been reading books, searching the Internet, and seeking a way to go through the "grief steps." Then the light bulb came on. My reality of losing Malachi and Hope was never going to change on this earth. No matter where I searched or how hard I tried, I was always going to miss them. I was always going to remember carrying, delivering, holding, and burying them. None of that would change. So I sat down in the waters. There weren't going to be any answers. In fact, it would be a lifetime of questions and wondering — a lifetime of my heart wondering what their personalities would have been like, what color their hair would have been as they grew older, what sports they would have liked, what they would have been gifted at doing for the Lord. At some point I realized that this is what I needed to do in my life. I came to this conclusion after Hope died. I am not quite sure when I chose this path, but in doing so, I have given myself the freedom to always miss Malachi and Hope.

No longer am I searching for a way out or for a way to get through the steps of grief. I have accepted these two amazing gifts; although I would do anything to change my reality, I have chosen to stop trying to search for a way out. I am allowing myself the freedom to grieve.

I don't know how this will look in the years to come, or even how it will look tomorrow. But I do know that my heart is free to always miss Malachi and Hope. By sitting in the waters everyone wanted me to be free from, I have allowed God to meet me and come sit with me.

Permission to Doubt
Allowing myself to be face to face with my heart has definitely brought some ugly truths to the surface. I see now that there are many ideas about God that I have believed without ever examining and there are many things I have made myself believe through the years. I did this without exploring the possibility of "the other side" of my heart. For example, God says in Hebrews 13:5, "Never will I leave you; never will I forsake you." I believed this to mean that God wouldn't allow things to happen beyond what I could bear because he wouldn't "forsake me."

While I never fully understood this truth, I always tried to will myself to believe it. It was said in the Bible so therefore I was going to believe it or else I wasn't a "good Christian woman." Who doubts or for that matter even challenges the Word of God? So I thought if the Lord allowed my children to pass away that meant I could handle it; and in that case, I had better be a good and faithful Christian woman and align my heart with His and accept my reality.

In therapy I eventually came to the place where I had to give myself "permission" to wonder why. It was so difficult for me to reach that place and allow myself to ponder all that was going on in God's plan. I had to give myself permission to entertain thoughts that even at times made God seem like He didn't know what He had done or was doing — thoughts that questioned the goodness of God in my life. I let myself be angry with Him. I let myself feel the pain of my deep sorrow.

It was ugly. It was a brutal place to go to. I lay down on the floor of my heart and allowed myself to have the greatest temper tantrum of all times. I wasn't in the place any longer in my walk with God that I could just "know His truths, accept, and believe." I had to actually believe it for myself. This is much like the difference between looking at a picture of the Grand Canyon versus standing there and seeing its beauty and grandeur for yourself. I know God now in a way that I didn't before I lost Malachi and Hope.

I would love to say that I am on the other side of this now. However, I am one stubborn girl. To this day, I have moments, even days, where I question God and all He has allowed. However, what is different now is that I know, truly know, His beauty and have seen His love for me in ways I never had before. I wouldn't have arrived at this place unless I would have accepted the journey.

It's fine with me if you can't understand this part of who I am. You don't have to wrap your head around it. This was between God and me. That's why we have a personal relationship with Him. My relationship won't look like yours. In my relationship, I had to arrive at the place where I knew what God had said in the Bible was true. It couldn't just be parts of it, because for me that isn't fully believing. I wanted to get to the place where I could hear the truths about God and His character and not cringe.

I wanted my heart to be in the place where I could hear a verse like Jeremiah 29:11, "'For I know the plans I have for you,' declares the Lord, 'plans to prosper you and not to harm you, plans to give you hope and a future.'" and actually believe it in my heart. I needed to believe that God is good — no matter what is happening in my life. I don't want to blindly accept those words any longer; I wanted to wholeheartedly believe them.

For me, this meant accepting the idea that a twelve-step program or a set of guidelines doesn't have to rule my grief. My grief looks more like a fine sewing pattern — where one color of thread ends and you see you are finished with that section, another color begins where you must start again.

While I now believe God is good and loves me, I know this doesn't mean I won't ever question Him again in this area of grief. I am actually certain I will question Him again. However, like all solid relationships, I know God can handle my wonder. I know He can handle my anger, my tantrums, and my inconsistencies. God wants me to truly believe in Him. His desire is that I would seek Him with my whole heart (Jeremiah 29:13). For me to honestly do this in my relationship with God, I had to get real with Him, and I have to stay real.

Your journey through your grief isn't going to look like mine. Sure, we will have threads that may be the same color, but the patterns of our hearts are unique. I encourage you to take the time to sit and question Him. Ask Him, why these colors? Why this fabric? Be honest and tell Him you hate the pattern! Trust me. I know you will find that your Father is creating you into a piece so creative and wonderful, and you would have never known unless you took the time to ask.

The kids talk about heaven and Jesus. They ask so many questions about what Jesus has in heaven. Whatever they ask me, I tell them that He has it because I want them to not feel scared about heaven. They seem to really understand.

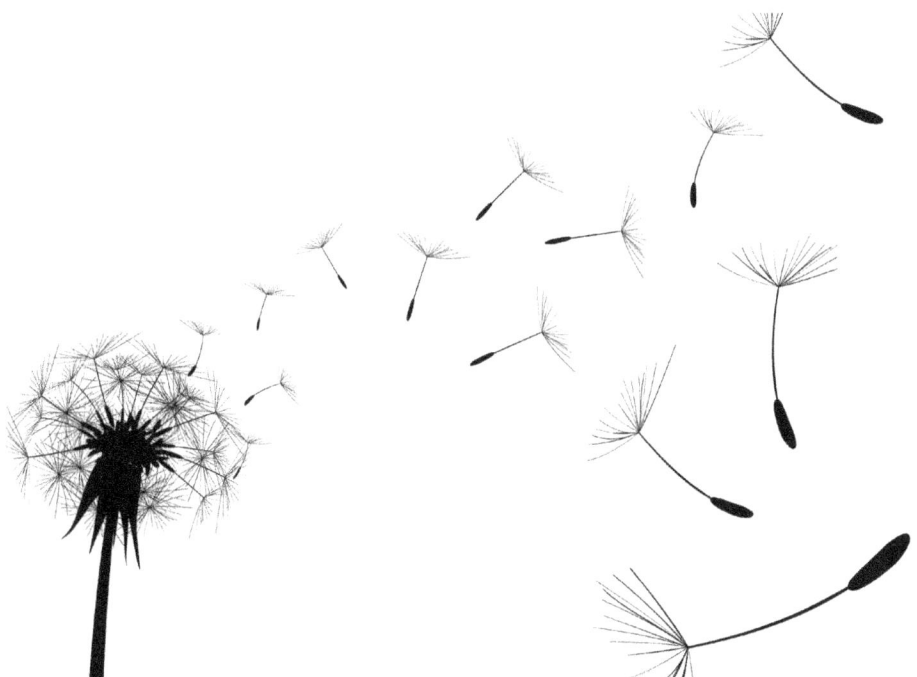

8

Letting Your Children Grieve

In this chapter I am going to take you through a few things we tried with our children as we all grieved. At the time of intense grief, our children were all quite young; the oldest was just six. Our suggestions and ideas are not based on professional advice. If you see that your living children are becoming withdrawn or cannot express their grief, I would seek professional help. We all need help at times in life. Do whatever you can to let them know you are supporting them, even if it is through an outside source. You might look for help through your church, your children's pastor, a counselor, or through services offered through your local city programs, which are often free. If you do not have the energy to find these avenues of help for your children, ask someone you love and trust to do this for you. It is critical they get the help they need as they are processing.

As our children have gotten older, they have expressed their grief differently. They aren't hesitant to talk about their brother and sister. If they have questions or just want to talk about them, they are quite open and have free rein. Their questions are bigger now. They ask more questions about why God allowed Malachi and Hope to go home. They want to hold them and don't understand why other kids get their siblings and they don't.

I don't have much to offer in the way of advice. What I have realized is that I can't fix their grief. So, I just sit down in their grief and mourn with them. I let them talk. I let them cry. I let them miss their siblings. I also make close friends, family, and teachers aware if they are struggling. They each have a journey with God. I have to trust He will carry them through.

It is probably clear to you by now that I don't exactly believe in the "grieving process." That said, I would like to share with you here how we have helped to lead our children through their grief. But first I must confess that we have made many mistakes. We have yelled at our kids. We have let out emotions when we should have held them in. We have missed opportunities to listen to them and comfort them. We have also missed times when we should have encouraged them and led them as they shared their grief with us. I am no expert in this area, but I can offer what I have learned through experience, and hopefully is will be helpful for you.

Grief is immensely challenging with children, and many times you have to think on your feet as you lead them. Often times, you only have a few minutes or even seconds to respond to their questions before they are off to the next thing. Don't beat yourself up if you "miss an opportunity." There will be more. None of us is a perfect parent. Fortunately, we have one who is. And He can meet our children where they are at any time. When we miss something, He steps in. When we mess up, He comes alongside them and lets them know *He* is their Savior.

Learning How *Your* Kids Grieve
With both Malachi and Hope we decided to have the post-funeral

gathering at our house. Many people offered to have it at their home for us. We declined because we really wanted to have it at our home. Our kids called the gathering "their party." They wanted people to come to their house and be with them. We had a select small group attend with each funeral. We took this approach because we felt we needed boundaries and so did our children.

The only children we allowed to attend were cousins. We asked other people attending to keep their children at home. We did this because our kids needed to be able to let their emotions out and feel safe. They also needed an outlet to vent. We weren't sure they would feel free to be emotional if they were surrounded by tons of kids. Our desire was to make certain their environment was constructed for them to grieve if they needed to. We had our pop-up pool set up for them and various people hung out with them while they played outside. We also played with them and made sure they knew we were right there for them. There are too many emotions, too many insurmountable concepts for a child to process in this day. So we tried to have fun things outside for them to do so they were able to release their energy and emotions. In my experience, kids need to have other things in place that they can do that allow them to step away from the utter sadness and overwhelming sorrow of those attending.

On this day, there is so much sorrow. The people they love and care for are visibly upset. This is difficult for a child. There needs to be some outlet to just be a child. They need to know they can cry or laugh and it is safe to do either (or both!). Do what you both feel works for your children and best meets their needs. If that means crying for a little and then playing a game, then let them. If it means allowing them to be angry (even if it includes yelling), then let them, and guide them in that process. Let them know they are not bad or wrong for their anger. Let them know that in future times when they feel that anger, they might be able to let it out in a different way. In my non-professional opinion, yelling is fine, as long as it stays about the person who died and the anger does not turn into something unhealthy.

Our kids all grieve differently and each one needs a varied response of grace from us. Here is what I mean: There was a time shortly after Hope died that my older son had an explosion. He had not cried much up to this point. We did not push his tears; we knew they would come. We were getting all the kids ready for bed. On a normal day, I would have thought his agitation was just because he was tired. However, given the circumstances, I knew it was much more. He was about to let it all out. And he did. He began to scream and cry and tell us how angry he was. He told us how he felt through tears and in anger. He conveyed his broken heart. He had held it all in; but in that moment, he was ready to let it all go.

This was a healthy outlet for him. Now, if he did this every day and this was the only way he talked about Malachi and Hope, we would be concerned. What he needed was a starting point. Death is too stressful for adults to grasp and wrap our hearts around. We cannot expect any more from our kids. Give your children the grace they need; they will let it out. If you are worried about them, then seek professional counsel. Do whatever it takes to allow them a healthy road to express their own grief. Let them feel they (and their grief) are safe with you. Let them know you are on their side.

As a parent, this is going to be exhausting. You and your spouse are in deep suffering and you still have to stay in touch with your children. All you may want to do is climb in bed and lie there all day. But as the days press on and life continues, you have to get up and make meals and get people dressed. Life doesn't stop for those who grieve.

Getting Creative

Even though you are thankful for your children and you want to help them in their grief, your body, mind, and spirit are in so much agony that it is draining to even stand. Nevertheless, you have to press on to help them. What we have found is that we have had to create opportunities for our children to express themselves. We have had times where we would just color. We would not ask them to draw anything specific. As they started to color, their hearts poured out. They would draw pictures of our whole family, and they would draw themselves with their siblings. They would draw themselves holding their brother and sister. They would also draw Christian and I holding Malachi and Hope.

Even now, they draw pictures of Malachi and Hope and give their drawings to us. Their pictures are still so powerful. There, on this little piece of paper, they have produced what their hearts are feeling. They work so hard and so diligently to produce this expression of their grief. They are always so proud of their pictures when they show them to us. They have these soft smiles on their faces, ones we don't see at any other time.

They ask many questions about heaven. They ask what Malachi and Hope are doing. When they ask about heaven and what their siblings are doing, I usually respond with this question, "Hmm, I wonder.... what do you think they are doing?" Immediately, they have a response. It is like they have been thinking about this and they have it all planned out in their heads. Their responses differ from one day to the next, but they often talk about how Malachi and Hope are playing. They are sure that Malachi and Hope are at the best creek ever. If they fall out of a tree, they won't be hurt. If they want to touch all the animals they find, they won't bite. They have even asked us if there is a Wii in heaven. Our answer was simple: "Yes, I bet there is a Wii in heaven. God has the best games ever!"

THE HEARTBREAK OF STILLBIRTH

We decided that we would help them to know that heaven is a place that God has prepared for us. He knows what we love and He wants to make it special for us. He has the best games, toys, and snacks we could ever dream of. We want them to feel that their brother and sister love where they are and are being perfectly cared for — which, of course, is true.

We really wanted to make sure the kids didn't feel that their little brother and sister were scared or lonely in any way. We did not want them to be afraid of heaven. We wanted them to know that Malachi and Hope are incredibly happy. We wanted them to know that Malachi and Hope want to be in heaven, that heaven is like home, and they want to stay there. When they have expressed their desires to hold them and let us know how much they miss them, we tell them we feel the same way. We reassure them that Malachi and Hope don't miss us the way we miss them. We tell them that they know a perfect love and a perfect Father. We explain to our kids that Malachi and Hope don't want to come home here on earth to be with us. They miss us, but they know that heaven is so much better than where we are. They know one day we will all be together. Malachi and Hope are not sad. They are so happy to be in heaven and they want to be there.

Our kids feel safe. They know that we step into their pain. We try to gently let them lead us in how they are feeling. We try to not put how we feel on them. We try to allow them to do the grief work that they need to do. The best conversations come seemingly out of nowhere. We will be talking about normal daily things, and then someone will say something like this: "If Malachi and Hope were in our van I know where they would sit. Malachi would sit with the boys in the back. Hope would sit next to Mathea in the front." It can be rather shocking and sometimes catch you off guard the way these things just pop up. Of course you have thought of these things as well, but somehow you think your kids don't think of such things. But they do. It may be different than how you feel it or in the timing that you experience it, but they do get there.

In these types of situations I usually want to cry. It would be fine if I did, but I also want to allow my kids to say more if they need to. My tears may prohibit them from saying what else is on their hearts. Sometimes they would say more and other times they would be on to the next thing so quickly. In this instance, my son proceeded to talk more about them and how cute they would be in the van. He asked how old they would be in relation to other babies he knew. It was so painful to sit through this conversation and to not break apart. But it was what he needed at the time. This is exhausting as a parent because you are grieving too. On the other hand, it is an incredible time to grow with your child. They get to experience a love that you are able to share with them that is so rare and so precious.

Working Through the Mistakes

Then there are the times you will miss the opportunity. Here is an illustration of a time I did. One night right after Malachi died, Christian had just gone back to work. Our lives had been turned upside down and now we were going back to "normal" life. He had left for a night meeting at church. My older son began to cry and then the others had their moments. I was not in the mood for this at all. I got the other kids to settle, but I couldn't get our older son to calm down. He cried for forty-five minutes. I tried being loving and understanding. Then as time wore on I tried to lay the law down. I got firm. I wanted to get everyone into bed. I was tired and knew he was as well.

He kept telling me that he didn't want "Daddy to die." I tried my best to reassure him but I could not promise that he would come home. Then I started to get annoyed at his tantrum. I knew it was all folded up in losing his baby brother, but I just wanted the kids in bed. His outburst was keeping everyone awake. I couldn't put the other kids to sleep while he was freaking out.

Eventually I said to him, "Daddy has to work. He has to go and make money. Do you know what happens if he doesn't work? We won't have any food, we can't pay our bills, and we will live in a cardboard box on the street. Do you want to live in a cardboard box?" Ugh. This probably has years of therapy for him written all over it. I can only pray that the Lord somehow uses that one!

I am sure the difference of how I handled both situations is strikingly clear. Of course, I had to say I was sorry to all of the kids. I had to settle him down and comfort him. My words were of no use. I let off steam. This wasn't just upsetting to him, but it made him feel insecure as well. Part of his tantrum was valid. The other part was just emotions that he had no control of because he is just a child. He hasn't learned all the ways of coping and how to let out how he feels. Sadly, I had no grace for it.

I look back and even though I still feel badly about what I said, very badly, I do find humor in it. I mean, who did I think I was? Chris Farley? "Livin' in a van down by the river!" I am sure if you've ever seen that comedy routine, it crossed your mind when you read my cardboard box story. I can only hope if my son remembers that night, he finds humor in it as well. Mostly I hope he doesn't remember it!

I do wish that I could go back to that night and just scoop him up and hold him. Just hold him until he was finished crying. But I can't go back. I just have to know that I messed up, and that Jesus will show Samuel that He is the only perfect Savior and Redeemer. I tell my kids all the time, "I am not perfect. If I were perfect, you wouldn't need Jesus. It is because of my total imperfection that you will run to Jesus. You will realize you 'need' a Savior. So, you have me to thank when you come to this conclusion." Of course, this is laced with humor. I am completely being sarcastic. The point of this joke is to tell them, "Hey, parents are not perfect. We don't want to, but we may hurt you at times. We just pray that Jesus will heal those places and restore you. We hope that our mistakes as earthly parents will help you see the perfect love of your Heavenly Father who doesn't make mistakes." I think this also makes kids feel safe. I mean, they can know they can mess up and it is all right. There can be forgiveness and still a healthy relationship in place. They can know the safety that comes from parents who love them and won't leave them.

So if you have messed up, know it is going to work out. Just ask forgiveness for the situation. Work it out. Then pray and ask the Lord to bring healing and comfort in a place where you failed. He is the Redeemer and He can bring good out of your mistake.

By doing this, you are inviting your children to be who they are. You are allowing them to know they can say what they need to say and not be judged. They can feel what they need to and know you still love them and are there for them. It is not always easy. Most of the time it is painful for you to hear their sorrow. As parents we naturally try to shelter our children from pain and sorrow. When the pain does come, there is nothing else to do but cry out to God and ask Him to lead you as a parent and trust that He will. He won't leave you or your children. Hosea 6:3 says, "As surely as the sun rises, He will appear." Praise the Lord that each day we can be assured that, "He will appear" in our lives and our children's lives.

Last night Christian was crying.
I mean, I cannot change this for him in any way.
He is hurting and I have to let his heart hurt.

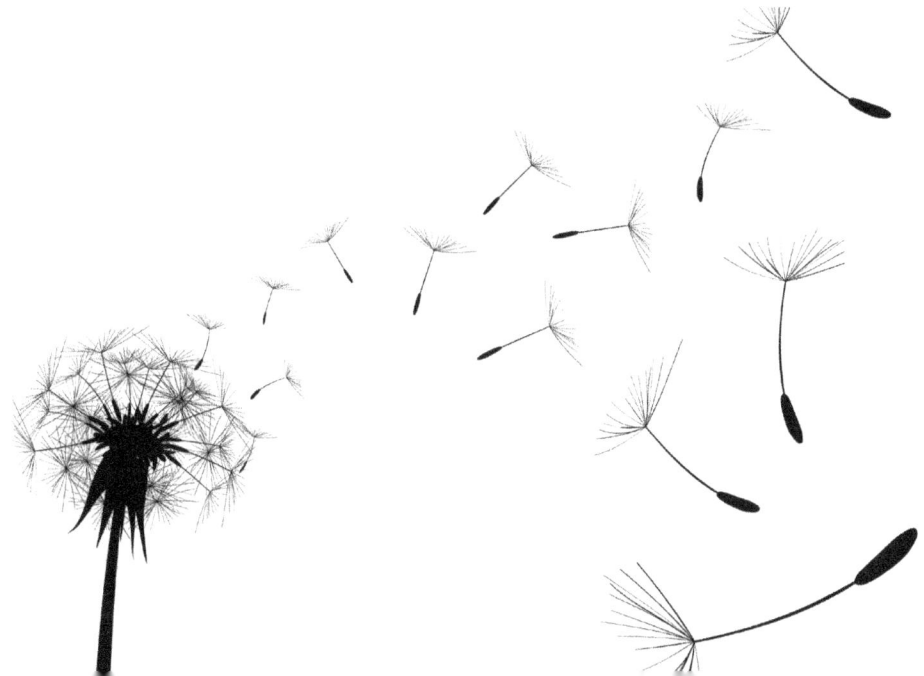

9

Grieving Together

Shortly after Christian returned to work, I called him, very upset. I was alone at home with the kids. I wasn't ready to be alone, but I didn't want anyone around either. I called him and started to vent. I told him how unfair it was that I had to be home surrounded by emotional kids, my own emotions, and the reality of life never stopping. I couldn't escape. I was angry that he got to go to work and talk to grown ups, try to distract himself, and even just be out of the house! The conversation escalated. He had to remove himself from a meeting. Finally, I had pushed his buttons so much, he threw his cell phone across the church parking lot and it imploded.

This is just one small illustration of the havoc grief can wreak on a marriage. Grief makes it easy to attack the people closest to you — to take out your pain on them. But there are other challenges as well. It can be difficult to accept your spouse's grieving process while you, too, are grieving. And of course, when you are in the midst of such pain, it is not easy to comfort others, even if that person is your spouse.

When there is such deep grief in your life, you will probably find that you need to learn new ways to support your spouse; the old ways just won't work. You will need each other in a way you never have before but you'll also feel like you have less to give than ever before. The unfortunate reality is that you cannot ease the pain of death.

This is a place in life where you have to rebuild your marriage from a new foundation. This is a terrible time for such fundamental changes. When a loved one dies, married couples struggle to come together. I have heard that death is one of the major reasons people get divorced, and I can understand why this happens. I feel that the Lord has given us such grace and mercy. I know we would not be where we are today without His intervention in our marriage.

When you are in agony, you want your spouse to come alongside you and aid you. But when your spouse is in the same agony you are in, so there is no one there to come alongside you. There is just a huge hole. You realize that you cannot carry your spouse. You realize that no matter what you do, you cannot take away their pain. You cannot lessen their pain. You sit there and hear them wailing, and not one word of comfort will satisfy their broken heart. You see them ripped to shreds and you ache inside. It is quite a hopeless feeling to see their tears, anger, and depression and to know that there's absolutely nothing you can do to ease their pain. There have been so many times I have awakened to Christian crying. I look at him and see that he is just crushed. So broken. So beaten down.

When your spouse is in this type of pain and you are as well, it seems like a river has come between you. You grieve differently. You process your pain and sorrow in different ways. This river can cause permanent separation if it is not dealt with. I know Christian and I had many good fights about our grief. What? Did you think that somehow we just fell in love all over again under such strain?

Ah, the stories I could tell you…I will spare you the details and leave much of it between us and God, but I can say that many colorful words were spoken and voices were raised. Fortunately, we made a good choice to only argue when the kids were asleep. We didn't want to put them in the middle of how we felt. We didn't want to make them feel insecure or cause them any more stress than they were already experiencing.

Sometimes during the day my anger would bubble beneath the surface and I would think to myself," I can't wait to talk to you about this later!" Ugh. Sounds so forgiving and Christ-like, right? Then at night there were times when I wanted to yell at Christian but knew I couldn't since the kids were upstairs sleeping. Instead I would make my face contort into something hideous and quietly seethe my words toward him.

What was all this fighting about? I am not actually sure I remember much of it. Thankfully, I don't. What I do remember was just knowing we were on different planes. We both were suffering the same loss but we were processing our grief differently. Yes, we felt the same sometimes, but how we expressed it or let it out was different most of the time. This is where it would get very challenging. You can't tell someone how to grieve. That is ridiculous. You can't say to someone, "Well, you aren't crying, so I guess you are feeling alright." That would be ludicrous. I see that now; at the time, however, I wanted Christian to grieve just like me. How you express your grief internally, externally, and within your relationship will most likely not be the same, but you want it to be. Reaching that place of understanding and accepting the differences in your expression and process of grief is where the struggle comes.

Eventually I came to see it like this: Christian and I were both in the same river, because we were grieving the same loss, but we each had our own way of getting to the other side. If you are feeling separated by your grief, one way to come together is to acknowledge that you're both in the same raging river. Remember what you have in common — the same waters are threatening you both — and then allow your spouse to navigate the river in their own way.

    I remember feeling at times that I wasn't "okay" and that Christian was processing his grief differently than I was. When life was back to "normal" as people say, he had to go to work. He had to resume parts of his life. I didn't have to do that in the ways he did. I was still home. Even though I homeschooled, my world did not change much from day to day. I couldn't escape the reality that I had gained fifty pounds. When I was able to exercise I would run in my neighborhood and cry. The weight was a constant reminder of how my body had changed for Hope, and now it felt like the sacrifice was in vain. My body was postpartum and I did not have my daughter in my arms. He did not have to deal with that reality. Getting dressed every day was not a challenge for him. Losing weight was not on his agenda. Dealing with post-partum emotions and hormones were not issues he struggled with. He didn't have to ice down his chest with bags of frozen vegetables because his milk was coming in.

    Immediately following a stillbirth, just the gender difference works against you. As a woman, you will struggle with physical issues and emotions your husband does not have to deal with. Christian was completely aware and compassionate toward the issues I had to deal with. There wasn't anything he was able to do for me to take away these difficulties. All he could do was watch me endure these trials and pray for me.

The Freedom to Pray
I think this is the next big step: realizing all you can do is pray for your spouse. Prayer feels inadequate in times like these. When life is so painful, it feels like there should be more we can do for the people we love. But

prayer is powerful. It goes beyond what we feel and what we desire for the person. Prayer has the power to touch God's heart. Prayer has the power to come into a situation and bring what we cannot offer. Prayer invites the Holy Spirit to come into our sorrow and comfort like only He can. Prayer has the power to bring peace, a peace that goes beyond the grave. This is where you can find common ground with your spouse. You are faced with the reality that there is nothing you can manufacture to bring about comfort. So you pray. By praying, you are asking the Lord to come and to touch the one you see in agony. You cannot take their sorrow away, but the Lord can touch their heart in ways that you are not able. For me, it was a point of surrender.

When we lost Malachi and Hope, I realized that any way that I had comforted Christian in the past wasn't going to work. I fell short. Eventually I realized that it was okay to not be able to comfort him and ease his pain, and that is when I could fully surrender him to the Lord. I could pray for him and ask the Lord to do what I was not capable of. Knowing this gave me freedom.

It is freeing to know that my prayers are what Christian needs from me. I am giving the Lord permission to work in his heart. I step out of the way and make room for Him. When I am not there to get in the middle, then the Lord can truly work His ways, which are always better than mine (Isaiah 55:9).

I think for so long I thought of prayer as second class. Prayer was good, but I felt I also needed to do something in the natural for the person I was praying for. But when there is nothing to "do," then I guess it falls to just praying, right? Through this time, the Lord began to show me just how powerful He can be when I surrender all and trust.

Maybe you are thinking, *That's it? Your advice is to pray?* Yes. That is my advice. If you are finding that you and your spouse cannot support one another in the ways that you once have, you don't know where to go from here, and you don't have the strength to figure anything out because your heart is broken — then yes, pray. Because when we invite the Lord in, He goes beyond our expectations. God "is able to do immeasurably more than all we ask or imagine, according to his power that is at work within us" (Ephesians 3:20). He can't take away all of our pain here on this earth, but if we give Him permission, He can make a way in our suffering and reveal Himself to us.

Working at It

Often times in grieving as a couple you just need permission to be different in your expressions of grief. While you most likely will express grief in various ways, do not forget to cling to one another. The enemy would love nothing more than to wreak more havoc in our lives. Grief is a perfect time for the enemy to come in and rob your lives and make more sorrow.

It's going to be challenging. Plain and simple. Both of you will have to work like never before at loving, serving, and accepting your spouse. However, it can be done. While it will take effort, it is the best thing you can do for yourselves and for your family. You will each have to lay down your lives for each other. When you do this, it opens the door for the love of God to come in and overwhelm your hearts for each other. Pray the Lord gives you compassion for your spouse. Pray He gives you ways to bless your spouse to demonstrate you care even if you can't understand where they are in their grief. For example, I absolutely love candy. I know it sounds ridiculous, but if I had a horrendous day, Christian would bring home candy for me. It was simple. It wasn't expensive and it was his way of saying, "I can't change it, but I love you."

There are of course other ways to show your love and to support your spouse. One important way is to give your spouse some time and space. There have been times since Malachi and Hope died that Christian has needed to get away in nature. It's one of his preferred ways of seeking God and being alone. It gives him time to journal, hike, be in nature, and listen to God.

Finding these avenues to bless your spouse will open the door for the Lord to work in your marriage. It's the daily choice to point your heart to God and ask for His wisdom in this area. He will lead you; He wants to lead you in your marriage. What we need to do is ask and seek Him.

There is a bond that comes when you allow the Lord to invade your marriage in the grieving process. If in the darkest hours of your lives you can expose your true thoughts and beliefs, then over time you will grow closer. I can honestly say Christian is my best friend. Time and time again he has shown me God's love by accepting and walking with me. In laying his life down for me he has created a safe place for me to express my heart, knowing he loves me no matter what. There is a bond that is made that is God given. When couples grieve and allow the Lord to invade their hearts together, He forms a bond that is truly given by grace and the power of His undying love for your marriage.

I want to encourage you in your marriage. Don't lose what you have. Take back the land the enemy has stolen and build on it. Find the help you need. Ask your pastors to pray for you and meet with you. Seek professional help for your marriage if you need it. We did. For many people the idea of "professional help" sounds scary. I mean, if you have reached the point of professional help, you must be truly messed up, right?

That's not at all how I see it. Counselors and therapists have the resources you do not have. It's like going to a doctor when you are sick.

THE HEARTBREAK OF STILLBIRTH

You can't prescribe yourself medicine when you are ill, can you? You have to seek help. I believe the same principle is applied in therapy.

It's not a place to complain or lay on a couch and be cross-examined. It's a safe place where you can talk without worrying about what others will think. It's a place of confidence, a place where you can share your pain and someone will be able to guide you both in your journey.

It is hard work. Therapy isn't time out of your day to just vent. Therapy is a place for you to grow. Often times, this means you will get homework. Let's face it, if we want to grow and bond with our spouses we have to work at it. But, it's worth it. It's worth the time and money.

Be willing to go to therapy even if you aren't crazy about the idea. If one spouse needs it more than the other, that is okay. It's just a season. Do your best to support the different avenues each of you may need to try.

I say all of this with a heart full of compassion. None of this is easy. Walking together in grief is completely challenging. The reward you will get by walking with one another is unexplainable.

I worry about what people will think — that we have "gone on" and that will never happen. The idea we would go through another pregnancy again? It would be so stressful. Emotionally, I am not even sure I have the strength to go through it.

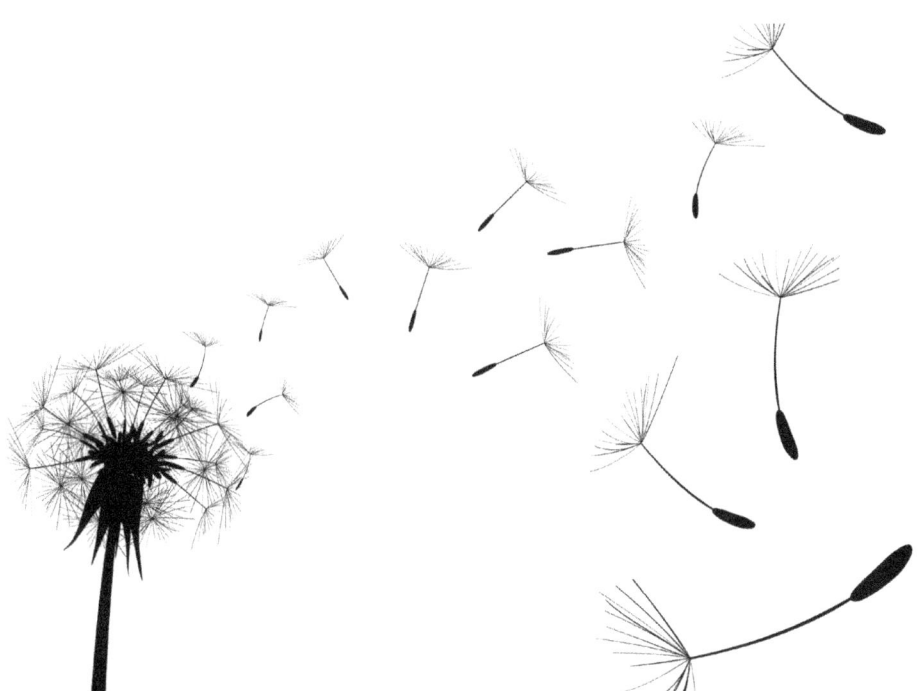

10

"Trying Again"

There is almost nothing I hate more than the phrase *trying again*. I hate the title of this chapter, but I purposely kept it to allow a perfect introduction to this chapter. (Please note my sarcasm.) This is the deal — *trying again* is such an awful phrase because it feels like the exact opposite of what it should be called. Couples should be able to grieve the loss of their baby without people asking them, "Do you think you will try again?" Whenever anyone asked me that, I wanted to rudely say, "Having another baby will not ease or take away my grief." Sometimes it almost felt as if people wanted us to "try again" so they wouldn't feel awkward around us, or so we could have a "good ending." (I get all fired up about this, let me tell you! Lucky for you (and me) I won't tell you half of the things I have wanted to say to people at times!)

This question almost feels like an offense. I am sure most people say this because they just don't know what to say. Or maybe they are curious and just want to know. For the most part, that question made me feel as if there was a disregard for our grief. It seemed to imply that in some way "trying again" would ease my pain. In this area of loss and death, I feel that "trying again" is a loophole for people to not truly deal with your pain and the horrible death of your baby. Trying again allows people to feel that one day you may "get what you wanted," or that you will not be as sad as you are now. The truth is that having another baby will not erase your pain. If you are able to have a living baby, that little one will bring you so much joy. However, that precious child cannot take the place of the one(s) you have lost.

A Decision Made for Us
I can write this with some experience. After Malachi died, we hadn't come close to making a decision as to whether we would consider having another baby or not. That decision seemed too difficult to have to make. To our surprise, we were blessed with the news that we were pregnant with Hope just five months after we lost Malachi. Her arrival was a sweet surprise, but it was also an emotional one.

We were in the midst of deep grief and suddenly our hearts needed to make room for joy and acceptance of another child. I fully believe that no matter how much you want the baby you are expecting, in the midst of happiness there can be some type of ambivalence. I felt so thrilled that she was with us. I felt so blessed by this sweet surprise from the Lord. But if I am to remain honest here, I also felt some ambivalence.

Those feelings haunted me. They served to compound my guilt and anxiety, and my feelings of being a failure as a mother. Suddenly, I was grieving *and* expecting — two opposite sides of the emotional universe. I couldn't just set aside my grief. That would have been impossible. I couldn't ignore the gift we had been given and only allow sadness to be her lot throughout my pregnancy with her either. I was forced to search deep within my heart and make room for both grief and joy.

When I took the pregnancy test and it was positive, both Christian and I cried. We cried because we were in shock. We cried because we were happy. We also cried because we were worried people would take this pregnancy as us "being ready" to have another child and walk this road. When people learned we were expecting, they started saying stupid things again. "This baby will bring you guys so much joy that you never got to have!" Or, "You must be so happy *now*!" The list goes on and on. Those comments can only make you laugh or want to hit the person. I suggest laughter!

If you do choose to try to have another child and become pregnant, what you really want people to say is, "Oh, I am so happy you are pregnant. At the same time, that must be so emotional for you both. You obviously will always miss your child. I will pray for you both." See? It isn't rocket science! Congratulations plus an acknowledgment of the child who is no longer with them.

I know it was hard for people to understand, but we were embarking on the most difficult journey of our lives. We were going to have to go to ultrasounds, appointments, get out the maternity clothes, and on and on. Each day we wondered if this new life would result in life or in more sorrow. In this time we felt so profoundly our need for others' prayers and compassion.

When I was pregnant with Hope, I didn't want to tell anyone until my first trimester was complete. I told Christian that I just could not deal with all of that yet. I wanted to wait until our first ultrasound so we could know that the baby was healthy. Christian was totally supportive. He did see wisdom in asking for prayer from people we trusted; however, he respected my feelings and all that I was going through.

Keep in mind the anxiety and depression that I was struggling through were in full swing and I just needed some space from people. I needed space from what people would say and how they would react. I didn't want to deal with other people's feelings and reactions when I didn't really understand my own.

I also felt protective of Malachi. I did not want people to assume because we had a baby coming that we had "moved on" or in some way that we were "ready." If you have lost, then you are familiar with these terms. You also know that it is impossible to "move on" or be fully "ready." Yes, your life keeps moving and you find new ways to live each day. However, there will always be a part of your heart that is set aside for the child you have lost.

At the end of the first trimester when we received the good news that Hope was healthy, we immediately told our kids and the rest of our family. As I mentioned already, we struggled throughout my pregnancy with what people would say to us. We realized that most comments were meant to comfort, but often it felt like pressure for us to just "be happy." It feels like our society doesn't deal well with death and grief. It is challenging for people to be around a grieving person. It is much easier to be around someone whose heart isn't in constant pain. It felt like many people were happy we were expecting, because they thought that would make us happy again.

So, will another baby bring you joy? Yes. Will the new little one bring happiness where there are tears? Sure. He or she may even bring emotions you didn't know were there. Your heart needs to be in a place of health and stability where you are able to process these emotions that will come. So how do you make this decision? How do you decide if you are going to try again?

The Path of Agreement

Personally I feel that agreement — your heart and your spouse's heart turned toward one another in unity — is where you must start before you walk this next part of your journey (if you are to walk it at all).

"Trying Again"

After we lost our daughter Hope, neither of us wanted to hear anything about "trying again" *again*. Sadly, this wasn't completely our choice. Once you have delivered your child, the testing as to why your baby died begins immediately. As you lay in the hospital bed recovering, they come to draw blood to start the testing. We could have refused a majority of the testing; however, we were compelled to try and learn what could have taken their lives. We wanted answers if there were any to be found.

Once they began the blood work, a flurry of testing followed. It was like a snowball effect. One test led to another and before we knew it we were immersed and our quest had begun. We did want answers; if there was a clear-cut one that could have been discovered quickly, why wouldn't we try and find out? Not that the answer would have lessened our grief at all, but it could have really helped in our search for what to do next. This is why we chose to continue pressing on with testing.

At first it appeared the answer could be right around the corner. However, after each test returned with no answer, the journey became laborious and painful. It wasn't as simple as going in for blood work. There were specialist appointments, insurance calls, and so many questions. Through all of this, our hearts ached. Going to these appointments meant exposing our hearts to many painful environments; we regularly saw pregnant women, newborn babies, fetal medicine specialists, and OB/GYN's. We were being thrust right back into a very raw and painful place.

I remember sitting in a waiting room shortly after delivering Hope and being surrounded by parenting, pregnancy, and baby magazines. What I would normally pick up and enjoy reading now made me feel totally sick inside. Christian and I would just hold hands and wait. Knowing we were in it together, we could silently support one another.

THE HEARTBREAK OF STILLBIRTH

That agreement we had was an anchor — like home base. When one of us would question the testing, we were able to return to why we had chosen this path: we were trying to find more answers. This is why I think it is so important in every step of the way to be in agreement as a couple. If you are not in agreement, then you won't be prepared for all that is set before you. It's so important to have someone to lean on through all of this.

At first, our reason for seeking medical answers was to research and find out if our living children were at any risk now or in the future. As the answers unfolded we began to see that there was a possibility for me to have a mild clotting issue. It was unlikely given I had never presented this issue before. However, as many of the doctors told us, nothing was out of the question. Some of the doctors we met with were humble and admitted that medical science can only determine so much; the rest, they said, was out of their control. Their advice was to keep pursuing medical answers and see where they would lead us.

We endured many weeks of stress while we waited for the results, but, thankfully, our genetic testing returned normal. Next we moved on to other specialists. Of course these involved weeks of waiting for appointments to open up, more testing, and more waiting for results. Basically, we went through about a year and a half of an emotional roller coaster, with many highs and lows. What would seem like good news would always end up in a negative light. Often the "high" of the seemingly good news would last a month or so, until we found out the rest of the story and were brought back down again.

Sure it seems normal that these highs and lows would take place. Life often makes us wait even though we wanted answers yesterday or a year ago. It all becomes different when you are the one waiting — when you are the one on the roller coaster.

"Trying Again"

If you are in the place of trying again, know that trying again will bring stress. Stress will come in places you expected and in places you never saw coming. This again supports my argument for being in complete agreement as a couple. If there is any hesitation for either person, this stress has the power to really make things difficult in your relationship.

For us, deciding to try yet *again* was not something we took lightly. We waited until all of our medical testing was done (which by and large was inconclusive) and worked in therapy for months (throughout the testing process) to find peace and agreement about which way to move forward. We also sought the Lord both together and on our own. We were praying together and asking for His guidance and leading in our lives. And even with all of this, we still felt at a loss for what to do. Finally, after months and months of this, our therapist thought it would be beneficial to take a block of time with the Lord on or own and think and pray for an extended period of time. Then, we could come back together and share what the Lord had shown each of us.

During my time with the Lord I went to the prayer room in our church. I walked in and had no idea what to do. I started to pray and then I just felt the Lord's leading to put some music on and just sit and wait. Only one CD appealed to me, so I played that. I hadn't ever heard the entire CD, and it almost felt strange that the music wasn't really comforting and familiar. Nevertheless, I sat there, closed my eyes, and listened.

The Lord brought to my mind the last time that I had been in this room praying. I sat there and cried as I remembered pleading with God for Hope's life. I remembered the desperation of our prayers. I spent a good amount of time going from crying to praying, and back again. Then the Lord had me really take note of a decoration in the room. I have seen this decoration a hundred times, but this time the Lord opened my eyes and had me see what this decoration meant for me.

It is a rustic cross with a miniature white rose bud tied to the middle of the cross by a vine of thorns. The Lord used this small cross to reveal to me His love for Malachi. At Malachi's funeral, we placed miniature white roses on his casket as we said good-bye. Here I was gazing at this very type of rose strapped to the cross. The rose was embedded and tied down, but it was living and beautiful.

I felt the Lord was speaking to me about His love for Malachi — how He died so Malachi would live forever. It was surprisingly comforting. In that moment, I was able to see how Malachi's life would live on here with me and our family and into eternity as well. It is a picture that will stay with me in my heart and keep speaking to me as the years go by. Much of my time there was very bittersweet. I was rejoicing that God was speaking to me about Malachi and Hope, and I was torn that my sweet children were not mine to keep. The Lord truly ministered to me in ways that were extremely personal in my grief and sorrow.

As I sat there and listened to this CD, I began to feel like I was ready to go home, that my time seeking the Lord was ending. I was ready to go and honestly I didn't know much about what God wanted me to do concerning our decision. I felt He had touched my spirit but I didn't have any sense of what was next for us. I got ready to leave and I felt the Lord tell me I needed to listen to one more song. So I sat back in the chair and another unfamiliar song came on. Here are the lyrics:

> *God moves in a mysterious way*
> *His wonders to perform*
> *He plants His footsteps in the sea*
> *And rides upon the storm*

"Trying Again"

Deep in unsearchable mines
Of never failing skill
He treasures up His bright designs
And works His sovereign will

Ye fearful saints, fresh courage take
The clouds you so much dread
Are big with mercy and shall break
In blessings, in blessings
In blessings on your head

Judge not the Lord by feeble sense
But trust Him for His grace
Behind a frowning providence
He hides a smiling face
His purposes will ripen fast
Unfolding every hour
The bud may have a bitter taste
But sweet will be the flower

Blind unbelief is sure to err
And scan His work in vain
God is His own interpreter
And He will make it plain

In His own time
In His own way...

THE HEARTBREAK OF STILLBIRTH

When I heard the verse about the bud, I opened my eyes and quickly sat up. What?! What had I just heard? I checked it again, listening to it so closely. Sure enough, the Lord had so sweetly placed this song to speak clearly to my heart. "The bud may have a bitter taste, but sweet will be the flower." In that moment, for the first time in two years, I felt like God was leading me. I felt like I had a path to move into. Part of me was terrified of all that trying again would mean for me and my family. The other part of me had this small glimmer of faith that I could find a place to stand. Hope came to me because God had spoken to my heart through this clear picture of the rose and the cross.

Later that night, Christian and I came together and recounted what God has shown each of us. In case you are wondering, I will briefly share what the Lord showed Christian. He actually did what all strong believers do — after praying and waiting for several hours, he finally said a quick prayer and whipped open his Bible, asking God to speak to him through the first verse he laid eyes on! When you are desperate, you'll do anything! Fortunately God is full of grace and can speak through even our feeble attempts, like throwing open our Bible — and He did speak to Christian that day. Christian opened his Bible to 2 Kings 4 and the story of Elisha and the Shunammite woman. Specifically he was struck by these verses (14-16): 'What can be done for her?' Elisha asked. Gehazi said, 'She has no son, and her husband is old.' Then Elisha said, 'Call her.' So he called her, and she stood in the doorway. **'About this time next year,' Elisha said, 'you will hold a son in your arms.'**

Pretty convincing right? Almost too easy. Even if it was "easy," Christian knew it wasn't a mistake and that the Lord had indeed spoken to him.

We talked that night after the kids had fallen asleep and shared with each other what had happened for each of us. Later we shared our

"Trying Again"

revelations with our therapist, and in her office we finally made our decision — a decision we'd wrestled with for so long and now we had an answer. We would "try again!" With this very emotional decision came relief over so many questions we'd struggled with for so long. As you might expect, the decision also came with a great amount of fear. Nevertheless, we had a path forward and we were determined to walk in it.

Because of our fear, we needed a list of parameters around our decision in order for us to walk along this path. We decided to try for three months and if I had not gotten pregnant, we would reconsider. This way we would ensure that our hearts could handle trying longer. Or we would decide that we were done, and ready to lay it down for good. To our surprise, we found out the very next month that I was pregnant.

We were shocked. I had never gotten pregnant so quickly. We both really felt that this was God's mercy on us. I also felt very ill prepared. Have you ever been on a roller coaster and at the end of it, it just stops abruptly and catches you off guard? That's pretty much how I felt. I was on this terrifying roller coaster trying to make a decision, going up and down, back and forth, around and around, and then finally it was done. I made the choice, and I was pregnant in one month! The ride had come to a screeching halt. Now it was time to start a whole new ride with its own twists and turns.

Having a living baby placed in my arms again was surreal. Watching her wiggle and squirm in those first moments of life felt like an out of body experience. So much joy that she was alive in my arms. The truth remains that no matter how amazing holding Eden was, her life didn't somehow make me forget holding my son and my daughter who had died. Each life is separate. Each birth is separate. Each story of their lives is separate. Earthly joy doesn't replace sorrow. I wait for the day when true joy wipes it all away. That cannot exist in, or be placed on, a person. It is up to Jesus. It is what heaven is all about. No pain. No sorrow.

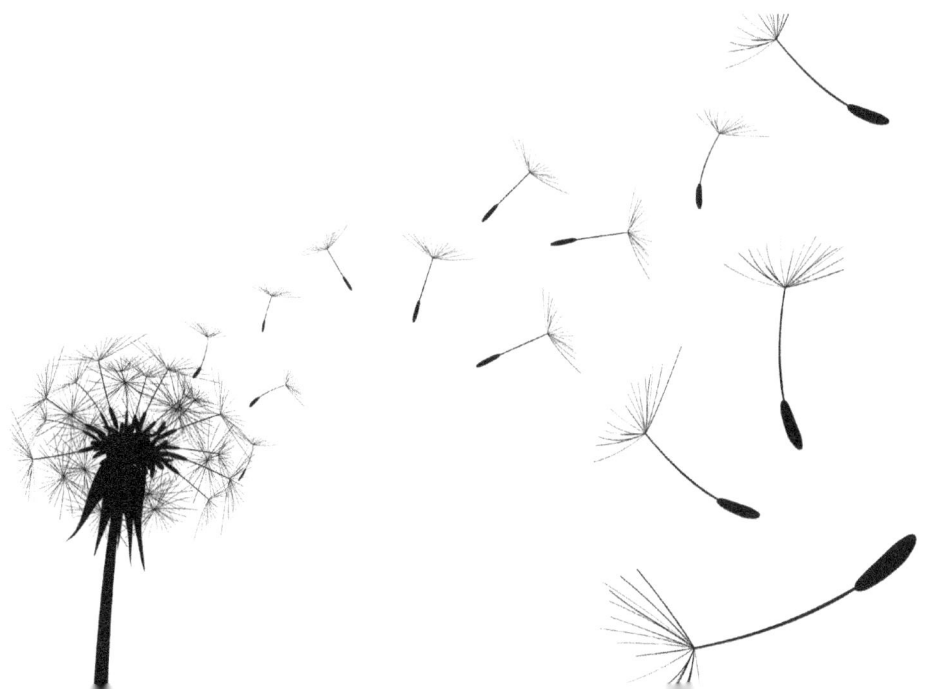

11

A Gift, Not a Substitute

Every person's journey is unique. I assume that your journey — like ours — includes the grief of losing a child to stillbirth, but I know that your journey before that moment and after will be different. Nevertheless, because I have shared so much with you, I would also like to share a bit about what it has been like for us to have a living child join our family after losing two children.

Holding our daughter Eden for the first time was incredible. She was moving. She was breathing. She was alive.

In a matter of minutes, however, our joy turned into terror when she was struggling to breathe. Of course it's not uncommon for babies to have trouble with those first breaths. But after Eden was born, aside from the standard attempts to engage and clear her lungs, she needed oxygen.

Of course I was worried, but I wasn't panicked. Not yet. She responded to the oxygen rather quickly and began to thrive on her own shortly after she received it. But about an hour later while I was nursing her, she turned blue. Literally blue. Not just her face. Her entire body was dark and discolored. We called the nurse in and I held her up; the nurse yelled, pushed the alarm on the wall, and screamed for help in the hallway. At this moment, the terror entered.

We had already called the kids, showed them a picture from the phone, and told them she was alive. Christian and I just stared at each other in disbelief. Looking over at the baby bed as they surrounded Eden felt all too familiar. We grabbed hands and began to pray.

She responded very well to the oxygen. However, there was no clear reason what caused her to suddenly turn blue and not breathe. Several pediatric doctors, including the head of pediatrics, came in to check her. They all suggested she stay an extra day and be monitored. Of course, we weren't leaving until she was monitored, so this was good news to us!

The adults in our families began to arrive after Eden was in good condition to receive visitors. At the time, there was a hospital policy that no child under twelve could visit due to the intense flu season, so our kids couldn't see their sister. They handled this exceptionally well, but it was disappointing for all of us.

It was wonderful to have family and friends come to meet Eden and hold her; they understood this was incredible yet emotional for us. All the same people who came to hold our children who had passed were now coming to hold our living daughter. This felt like a rollercoaster of emotion, acknowledging that there was now life and celebration in a place that had meant death and devastation. I was so grateful to have people there with us who understood that.

Delivering Eden and being with her in those first hours was a very raw experience. There I was, so thrilled she had arrived. I was snuggling her and kissing her, and I was barely willing to let go. My excitement was through the roof. At the same time, I was crying. Not just the normal tears from a very tired new mama. I was crying because there I was dressing my daughter in the outfit we had bought her and she was alive. There are no words to describe how that felt. Her hands were responding to mine. I was looking into her eyes and she was trying to open those new puffy eyes to look at me. Hadn't I just been here? Hadn't we just dressed Malachi and Hope in the clothes we had chosen for them? Held their hands? Kissed them?

In those days we stayed at the hospital, Christian and I had many times of worry that our daughter would die and many moments of joy for her life. There wasn't much level ground. How could there have been? We were high and low at each moment.

The kids responded with many of the same emotions, but it just looked different. They were amazing when we brought Eden home. I remember their sheer joy as we walked through the door with her. That moment was incredibly difficult for me. I had come home after delivering Malachi and Hope from the same hospital with nothing but pictures and baby blankets.

The kids couldn't wait to hold her. It was almost impossible to wait their turns. They couldn't kiss her or hold her long enough. Their faces beamed with joy over their sister. It was completely precious to watch. They took in every detail about her. " Mom! Look at her little eyebrows!" "Look at her tiny fingernails!" " I love the way her breath smells, Mom!"

Of course, Eden's life didn't erase their pain. Even now, we entertain deep questions about their brother and sister. Why they died. Why they can't hold them now. They have conversations with us about the sports Malachi and Hope would play, who they would be in school with, where they would sleep. The list goes on and on. We just roll with their questions and thoughts, and we let them do the same. We didn't have anything scripted or thought out to help them express their questions or emotions. Part of the reason we didn't prepare for any of these questions was because in our journey we had come to the place where we felt we had to just let it happen naturally. We didn't want to force them to "feel" certain things. We didn't want them to think they had to feel certain ways with Eden's arrival. We just decided to let it ebb and flow.

Joy and Questions

I know that many people who know us or our situation have thought that having another child would ease our suffering. I can only chuckle at this idea. A living child does not and could never replace your child who has died. It's just not possible. People want this to be true. People want this to be true so they can believe that you "get" something that is good. They want your story to have a happy ending.

This approach reminds me of Job. Job was stripped of all that could possibly be taken from a human — family, friends, health, and possessions. The Book of Job concludes with God blessing Job — restoring him above and beyond for his faithfulness to God. While Job "gets" all these "things" back, the lives of his dead children are of course not returned to him. Yes, he "gets" more children, but they didn't replace the ones he lost. He didn't just forget all he had suffered. He didn't forget his children and the horror he had endured.

This is how this idea resounds in my heart. I see all the joy and wonder Eden has brought into my life and the life of my family, but she doesn't take away the sting of burying Malachi and Hope. Please hear me: She gives me such joy. However, I will always miss Malachi and Hope. I will always cry when I remember their sweet hands and adorable faces.

Eden has brought laughter and joy to our home. Her life has also brought more questions for us to navigate through in our own hearts and as parents. I have questioned God about why Eden was allowed to live

A Gift, Not a Substitute

and my other children were not. Of course I love that she is here, but I have to ask, "Why not my other children?" It's part of the process for me. Being honest with God and letting myself explore these areas allows me to have a deep and real relationship with God. It may look different for you, and that is okay. But this is the way for me.

In many ways having Eden made me realize all the things I never got to do, or never will get to do, with Malachi and Hope. The losses became even more glaring. It was all there in my mind before, but now actually doing these things with Eden has made it very real. All of it. I have nursed her, diapered her, washed her clothes, made doctor appointments, and stayed up all night with her. I've heard her cry and laugh, and I've watched her learn to crawl, walk, and talk. All the things that I wanted to do with Malachi and Hope I have done with Eden. While it is amazing and I love being able to do these things with her and for her, it has been painful.

There is an obvious age gap in our family. To an observer, Eden might look like the "surprise baby." Or the baby we waited to have until we got past a few crazy years of little ones. There is a pattern to our family that not everyone is aware of. To people at the mall, in stores, or even at church, we appear to be one happy family. And while in many areas this is true, there are parts of our hearts that are quiet with pain.

Every day I see all the things I am missing with Malachi and Hope. I watch my sisters' children go to school in the grades Malachi and Hope would be in, and I see the sports they play and the funny things they do, and I miss my kids. I see other children grow, experience childhood milestones like losing teeth, and I wish my kids were here doing those things. All of these things make me miss my Malachi and Hope. I miss them in a way that is almost indescribable.

Yes, it is true we get to watch Eden do these things, and that is amazing. I don't take for granted all the wonderful life she brings to our home. Eden's life is a precious gift. There is no question about that. However, her life doesn't have the power to replace any of her siblings. Her life isn't meant to heal my heart. That isn't her role in this life, and it is not why God created her. Plain and simple: her life is a gift. I am happy for Eden that we are emotionally healthy enough to realize this. We wanted this little girl with no strings attached.

I feel like my thoughts and emotions bounce back and forth like a ball on a ping pong table. I go from being so thankful on one side to bouncing to the other side of grief. I don't want to play the role of a victim where all of life is horrible and one bad thing leads to another. I do see Eden's life as a treasure. How could I not? However, I also choose to be honest with myself and give myself permission to have these feelings about Eden and my family. I think it is important to allow yourself to face what your reality is and deal with what is in your heart. I fully believe if you don't do this, other life situations or trials will bring them to the surface.

I encourage you to always face your grief head on. Allow the truth to sink into your heart. This way you can be honest with yourself and the Lord. My hope and prayer is that you will allow the Lord to enter into this part of your life and that He will show you His grace and love.

www.ingramcontent.com/pod-product-compliance
Lightning Source LLC
Chambersburg PA
CBHW020003050426
42450CB00005B/295